SUBSCRIPTION INFORMATION

Annual Institutional Subscription, Volume 3, 2009

Institutions (print and online)	£222.00 (UK)	€318.00 (Europe)	$399.00 (RoW)
Institutions (online only)	£211.00 (UK)	€302.00 (Europe)	$379.00 (RoW)
Individiuals	£80.00 (UK)	€114.00 (Europe)	$140.00 (RoW)

Discounts are available for members of the following societies: International Society for Augmentative and Alternative Communication; Royal College of Speech & Language Therapists; Speech Pathology Australia.

Please email journals@psypress.com for details.

Subscriptions purchased at the personal (print only) rate are strictly for personal, non-commercial use. The reselling of personal subscriptions is prohibited. Personal subscriptions must be purchased with a personal cheque or credit card. Proof of personal status may be requested.

Dollar rate applies to all subscribers outside Europe. Euro rates apply to all subscribers in Europe, except the UK and the Republic of Ireland where the pound sterling rate applies. All subscriptions are payable in advance and all rates include postage. Journals are sent by air to the USA, Canada, Mexico, India, Japan and Australasia. Subscriptions are entered on an annual basis, i.e., January to December. Payment may be made by sterling cheque, US dollar cheque, euro cheque, international money order, National Giro, or credit card (Amex, Visa, Mastercard).

Subscription and single issue ordering information

Customer Services, Taylor & Francis, Sheepen Place, Colchester, Essex CO3 3WQ, UK. Tel: +44 (0)20 7017 5540. Fax: +44 (0)20 7017 4614. E-mail: tf.enquiries@tfinforma.com

Aims and scope

Evidence-based Communication Assessment and Intervention (EBCAI) brings together professionals from several disciplines to promote evidence-based practice (EBP) in serving individuals with communication impairments. We target speech-language pathologists, special educators, regular educators, applied behavior analysts, clinical psychologists, physical therapists, and occupational therapists that serve children or adults with communication impairments. We select and appraise the latest and highest quality studies and reviews related to assessment, intervention, diagnosis, and prognosis published across 60+ professional journals in speech-language pathology and related fields. We make these appraisals accessible through value-added structured abstracts that include expert commentary about the quality of the evidence as well as its practical implications. This affords the practitioner a one-stop reading experience to stay on top of research findings in order to facilitate evidence-based decision-making. Researchers and university professors will benefit from access to cutting-edge and clinically relevant studies.

EBCAI also provides a forum for the dissemination of original research and discussion of methodologies and concepts that advance EBP as well as of experiential accounts of relevant stakeholders involved in the EBP process.

Submissions: Please consult the Information for Authors for the specific kinds of submissions *EBCAI* seeks to publish. This can be found on the Journal's website at **www.psypress.com/ebcai**.

References should follow the APA Style Manual (5th ed.). Common examples:

Journal article

Schlosser, R. W., Wendt, O., & Sigafoos, J. (2007). Not all systematic reviews are created equal: Considerations for appraisal. *Evidence-Based Communication Assessment and Intervention, 1*(3), 138–150. doi:10.1080/17489530701560831.

Chapter in a book

Meltzer, P. S., Kallioniemi, A., & Trent, J. M. (2002). Chromosome alterations in human solid tumors. In B. Vogelstein & K. W. Kinzler (Eds.), *The genetic basis of human cancer* (pp. 93–113). New York: McGraw-Hill.

Evidence-Based Communication Assessment and Intervention (USPS permit number pending) is published quarterly (in March, June, September and December), by Psychology Press, 27 Church Road, Hove, BN3 2FA, UK. The 2009 US institutional subscription price is $399.00. Periodicals postage paid at Jamaica, NY by US Mailing Agent Air Business, c/o Worldnet Shipping USA Inc., 149-35 177th Street, Jamaica, New York, NY 11434. **US Postmaster:** Please send address changes to *Evidence-Based Communication Assessment and Intervention* (TEBC), Air Business Ltd, c/o Worldnet Shipping USA Inc., 149-35 177th Street, Jamaica, New York, NY 11434.

Back issues: Psychology Press retains a three year back issue stock of journals. Older volumes are held by our official stockists: Periodicals Service Company (http://www.periodicals.com/tandf.html), 11 Main Street, Germantown, NY 12526, USA to whom all orders and enquiries should be addressed. Tel: +1 518 537 4700; Fax: +1 518 537 5899; E-mail: psc@periodicals.com

Disclaimer: Psychology Press makes every effort to ensure the accuracy of all the information (the "Content") contained in its publications. However, Psychology Press and its agents and licensors make no representations or warranties whatsoever as to the accuracy, completeness or suitability for any purpose of the Content and disclaim all such representations and warranties whether express or implied to the maximum extent permitted by law. Any views expressed in this publication are the views of the authors and are not the views of Psychology Press.

The print edition of this journal is typeset by Glyph International.

The BMJ Publishing Group grants permission for the Pictograms to be reproduced in this publication, with non exclusive world rights in print and electronic formats.

Evidence-based Communication Assessment and Intervention
2009, 3(4), 191–194

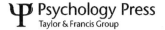

Introduction

Teaching evidence-based practice: An impetus for further curricular innovation and research

Ralf W. Schlosser[1] & Jeff Sigafoos[2]
[1]Department of Speech-Language Pathology and Audiology, Northeastern University, Boston, MA, USA, and [2]College of Education, Victoria University of Wellington, Wellington, New Zealand

Keywords: *Evidence-based practice; Academic training; Teaching methods; Undergraduate curriculum; Graduate curriculum; Clinical practice.*

Several national professional organizations of speech-language pathologists have adopted evidence-based practice (EBP) as the preferred approach to clinical practice. This mandate brings with it an added responsibility for university programs because they need to prepare future generations of speech-language pathologists for these new demands. We welcome our readers to this special issue on teaching EBP. We believe it is the first in a peer-reviewed journal in the field that focuses on the teaching of EBP at the pre-professional level.

Authors representing four university programs from three continents (Australia, Europe, and North America) showcase how they conceptualized and implemented innovative approaches to teaching EBP. Because many programs are in the midst of moving toward EBP, this special issue is timely for anyone who is teaching or learning in a university-based program in speech-language pathology or related field involving communication assessment and intervention.

It is our pleasure to introduce each of the papers. First, we have a contribution from the

University of Newcastle, United Kingdom. Dr. Thomas Klee (who is now at University of Canterbury in New Zealand), along with Drs. Stringer and Howard, shared how they have conceptualized and implemented EBP in their curriculum for speech and language therapy students (Klee, Stringer, & Howard, this issue 2009). They share their experiences in introducing EBP into the undergraduate curriculum[1] through an EBP-focused module as well as through clinical placement. The introduction of a module was timed to allow the swift introduction of EBP into the curriculum without major changes (that are possibly more time-consuming) to the other aspects of the curriculum. Readers will undoubtedly benefit not only from the authors' conceptualization of the module, but also their reflections on what seemed to work and what could be improved. Newcastle's innovative introduction of EBP into clinical placements is a necessary, but often neglected aspect (probably because it is more complicated) of teaching EBP at the pre-service level. The authors also share their experiences on implementing EBP to already practicing speech-language pathologists through a post-certification training program.

The second paper by McCabe, Purcell, Baker, Madill, and Trembath (this issue 2009) describes the approach taken by the

For correspondence: Ralf W. Schlosser, Department of Speech-Language Pathology and Audiology, Northeastern University, 151C Forsyth, Boston, MA 02115, USA. E-mail: r.schlosser@neu.edu

Source of funding: No source of funding reported.

faculty at the University of Sydney, Australia. Their model involves the use of a case-based approach to learning and teaching curricula in speech-language pathology at the undergraduate and master's level. The authors provide convincing rationales as to why case-based learning presents a natural fit for the teaching of EBP. In addition to sharing their experiences, they also present preliminary findings from an evaluation of the approach by students and instructors.

The third paper by Proly and Murza (this issue 2009) from the University of Central Florida describes an approach to teaching master's-level and doctoral-level students how to conduct systematic reviews. Systematic reviews are indeed one of the preferred evidence-based information sources. The authors eloquently persuade readers that the ability to conduct and use systematic reviews is critical to the implementation of EBP. Although their approach is focused on the production of systematic reviews, students who know how to carry out systematic reviews may acquire an appreciation for using systematic reviews once they enter clinical practice. It is probably safe to assume that most master's-level training programs rarely expose their students to the mechanics of producing systematic reviews. The curriculum developed at the University of Central Florida has successfully tackled this issue and continues to develop capacity in the field for EBP.

Last but not least, the paper by Raghavendra (this issue 2009) describes a master's-level EBP course in the speech-language pathology curriculum at The Flinders University of South Australia. The course is conducted as a 3-day intensive workshop and utilizes a problem-based learning format with a heavy emphasis on the use of research evidence through the development of critically appraised topics. The author shares important initial reflections based on student feedback and insights gained by the instructor.

Collectively, the papers provide an excellent read into the very practical issues involved in integrating EBP into existing speech-language pathology programs. We, as editors, have gained inspiration and numerous ideas for the development of our own EBP curricula at our respective institutions and we are confident that our readers will gain similarly from this special issue. In the remaining paragraphs, we would like to raise issues for future consideration as we move forward with developing or refining our EBP curricula in speech-language pathology and related fields. Please note that the issues are not arranged in any particular order such as priority or importance.

What is the evidence-base for the teaching methods chosen for our EBP curricula?

In addition to a conceptual fit, the teaching method selected should be efficacious. There may not be evidence inside our own field, but perhaps we can borrow from other fields.

Can we learn from related fields?

The field of speech-language pathology was among the allied health fields that adopted EBP more gradually than others such as physical therapy, nursing, or occupational therapy. These fields have had to contemplate the teaching of EBP in their pre-professional curricula before we have (e.g., Levin & Feldman, 2006; Slavin, 2004; Stern, 2005). Hence, it may be worthwhile to learn from these other fields in order to gain ideas and insights that we can adapt to our needs or, if nothing else, to avoid making the same mistakes that they may have made. Somehow, the discourse of EBP in the field seems to connect to the original source in medicine (which is essential), but never seems to step sideways to other allied health fields. In doing so, we may be missing out.

How can we ensure that EBP is taught in a way that is realistic?

University programs have the luxury to do things somewhat differently than is possible in the clinical practice setting. For many reasons, this is important because it allows for establishment of foundational skills in a safe and non-threatening environment. When EBP is taught, however, without being cognizant of the real practical constraints that practicing clinicians face on a daily basis (e.g., in terms of dedicated time, knowledge and skills, resources), we are setting our future graduates up for failure down the road. Our pre-professional curricula must help students anticipate these challenges and successfully cope with them. Or as Stern (2005, p. 157) put it,

> If we do not give voice to these realities, we run the risk of perpetuating yet another form of the "theory–practice divide."

How can we make sure that practicing clinicians also gain knowledge and skills in EBP?

While the main focus of the special issue was on teaching EBP in pre-professional curricula, it is critically important that practicing clinicians also gain knowledge and skills in EBP. When newly graduating speech-language pathologists and related professionals enter the workforce and find that EBP is not used in the field, they will find it hard to sustain their newly acquired knowledge and skills. The University of Newcastle program described by Klee and colleagues (this issue 2009) has recognized and found a way to involve clinical supervisors in their EBP training efforts. We need to develop more such efforts if EBP is to gain a foothold in day-to-day clinical and educational practice.

These are just some of the issues that require attention in the field. There is also a need to promote further curricular innovation as well as a need to conduct research on the effectiveness of these approaches. Given the importance to the field, it would seem that national organizations such as the Royal College of Speech and Language Therapists, Speech Pathology Australia, and the American Speech-Language-Hearing Association and international associations (e.g., International Association of Logopedics and Phoniatrics) should play a more active role in stimulating further curricular innovation and funding urgently needed research. It is our hope that this special issue may provide an impetus for these developments. With that in mind, we would like to thank all of our contributors not only for their efforts in shaping EBP curricula in pre-professional programs but also for putting it in writing!

NOTE

1. The undergraduate program in the UK is in many ways equivalent to what might be taught in master's programs in the USA.

REFERENCES

Klee, T., Stringer, H., & Howard, D. (2009). Teaching evidence-based practice to speech and language therapy students in the United Kingdom. *Evidence-Based Communication Assessment and Intervention, 3*, 195–207.

Levin, R., & Feldman, H. (2006). *Teaching evidence-based practice in nursing: A guide for academic and clinical settings.* New York, NY: Springer Publishing Co.

McCabe, P., Purcell, A., Baker, E., Madill, C., & Trembath, D. (2009). Case-based learning: One route to evidence-based practice. *Evidence-Based Communication Assessment and Intervention, 3*, 208–219.

Proly, J. L., & Murza, K. A. (2009). Building speech-language pathologist capacity for evidence-based practice: A unique graduate course approach. *Evidence-Based Communication Assessment and Intervention, 3*, 220–231.

Raghavendra, P. (2009). Teaching evidence-based practice in a problem-based learning course in speech-language pathology. *Evidence-based Communication Assessment and Intervention, 3,* 232–237.

Slavin, M. D. (2004). Teaching evidence-based practice in physical therapy: Critical competencies and necessary conditions. *Journal of Physical Therapy Education, 18,* 4–11.

Stern, P. (2005). Holistic approach to teaching Evidence-Based Practice. *American Journal of Occupational Therapy, 59,* 157–164.

Evidence-based Communication Assessment and Intervention
2009, 3(4), 195–207

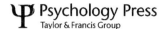

Psychology Press
Taylor & Francis Group

Teaching evidence-based practice to speech and language therapy students in the United Kingdom

Thomas Klee[1], Helen Stringer[2], & David Howard[2]
[1]Department of Communication Disorders, University of Canterbury, Christchurch, New Zealand, and
[2]School of Education, Communication and Language Sciences, Newcastle University, Newcastle, UK

Abstract
We outline three ways in which evidence-based practice (EBP) is formally embedded into the curricula for pre-registration Speech and Language Therapy students and experienced Speech and Language Therapists at Newcastle University in the United Kingdom. We describe key features of an undergraduate module, an undergraduate clinical placement, and a new Master's degree program, each aimed at encouraging critical thinking and clinical problem-solving skills in students.

Keywords: Education; Academic training; Teaching methods; Instructional model; Active learning; Evidence-based practice.

In this paper, we describe our experience of introducing evidence-based practice (EBP) into the undergraduate curriculum at Newcastle University in the United Kingdom. We outline two distinct aspects of how EBP has been embedded into the curriculum—one involving an undergraduate module (i.e., a course) and the other involving a clinical placement. We then summarize a new post-qualification (i.e., post-certification) Master's program, which is aimed at introducing the principles and practice of EBP to experienced Speech and Language Therapists (SLTs) for the purpose of developing their clinical research skills. The main aim of the new postgraduate program is to enable experienced SLTs to learn a new set of clinical knowledge and research skills or build on and further develop an existing set of skills. Another aim of the new postgraduate program is

For correspondence: Thomas Klee, Department of Communication Disorders, University of Canterbury, Private Bag 4800, Christchurch 8140, New Zealand. E-mail: thomas.klee@canterbury.ac.nz

Source of funding: No source of funding reported.

to provide a well-rounded, substantive foundation year for those wishing to continue into a PhD program, while stimulating others to consider pursing a PhD who might not otherwise have done so.

Newcastle was the first university in the United Kingdom to award a degree in Speech and Language Therapy, in 1967. Currently, two degree-level programs are offered for the purpose of training students to become SLTs; each is recognized by the Health Professions Council (the United Kingdom's regulatory body) and the Royal College of Speech and Language Therapists as a university qualification that leads to a license to practice as an SLT. The BSc in Speech and Language Sciences is a four-year undergraduate degree, and the MSc in Language Pathology is a two-year postgraduate degree. Successful completion of either degree allows graduates to apply to register as an SLT with the Health Professions Council. In this paper we focus on how EBP is currently embedded within the undergraduate program.

Both degree programs underwent a major review in 1999, resulting in changes to both

http://www.psypress.com/EBCAI   DOI: 10.1080/17489530903399103 their content and delivery. Among these changes was a pedagogical shift away from lecture-based modules to ones that employ case-based problem solving (Whitworth, Franklin, & Dodd, 2004) and an increased emphasis on developing students' research skills and applying research outcomes to clinical practice. Regarding the latter, students are required to take a series of research methods modules during the first three years of the program and conduct an empirical research investigation in their final year. The research project, known as the BSc dissertation, is the equivalent of the Master's thesis that is undertaken at some universities in the United States of America in fulfillment of a degree in speech–language pathology. In what follows, we outline various aspects of how EBP has been formally implemented at Newcastle: in an undergraduate module, in an undergraduate clinical placement, and in a new Master's degree program.

THE UNDERGRADUATE EBP MODULE

The curriculum of Newcastle's BSc program has always had a strong emphasis on theory and research, with these forming the foundation for training students in clinical practice. Consequently, clinical training is informed by theoretically motivated interventions and, where possible, by empirical evidence supporting the use of such interventions. In 2005, however, teaching staff recognized the need to go beyond this by finding a way of equipping students with the tools and knowledge required to conduct evidence-based assessments and interventions after graduation. This is not to say that students were ill equipped to engage in EBP before that time, but we felt what was needed was a way of distilling and presenting information in such a way that students would feel comfortable and confident in seeking out new knowledge and keeping up with developments in the field once they left university.

Equally important was the need to foster an attitude in students that led them to question, in a constructive and positive way, the things they were doing in clinic and challenged them to think in new ways for the benefit of their clients. One way of doing this was to draw together the three strands of the curriculum, involving academic, clinical, and research modules, in such a way that students could more clearly see the link among them—and see that each was important to the other if clinical services were to be delivered effectively. Thus was born a module specifically devoted to the topic of EBP.

Newcastle first offered a module called *Evidence-Based Practice in Communication Disorders* during the 2005–2006 academic year. The module was taught as a final-year option to undergraduate students as well as to students on the former MSc in Human Communication Sciences. The module was offered as a final-year option for two reasons. It was considered to be the fastest way of introducing new course material without investing large amounts of staff time changing other parts of the curriculum in order to accommodate the new subject matter, but, more importantly, it was felt at the time that having a single, coherent, and focused module would be the best way of ensuring that the material was learned.

When the module was first proposed at a staff teaching away-day, not only did someone volunteer to teach it, but three people did. With two people having an interest in developmental disorders and the third in adult disorders, we decided to collaborate in planning and teaching the module. The interest and enthusiasm for the new module was so high that all three staff participated in each and every class session—a situation that could have been overwhelming for the students, but fortunately did not appear to be.

Because the module was offered to students as an option, they had a choice of whether to enroll or not. We feared that some might perceive the module as being another research methods course, and, indeed, some who chose other options did voice this concern. So, to set the right tone and entice students to sign up, we suggested they read Goldacre's (2008) entertaining book about health research and how its findings are reported in the press.[1]

And, so that the module would appear inviting and nonthreatening, the opening paragraph of the syllabus read:

"Evidence-based practice is the conscientious, explicit and judicious use of current best evidence in making decisions about the care of individual patients" (Centre for Evidence Based Medicine, Oxford University, http://www.cebm.net). Having its origins in the fields of medicine and clinical epidemiology, EBP is now a growing part of speech and language sciences. Since 2003, speech and language therapists practising in the UK have been required to "be able to conduct evidence-based practice" (*Health Professions Council, 2007*). As Greenhalgh (2001) expressed in her book, *How to Read a Paper*, we hope this module will "demystify the important but often inaccessible subject of evidence-based medicine" (p. xii) and build on your previous knowledge in this area by introducing you to ways of judging the value of assessment procedures and intervention practices in speech and language sciences.

The purpose of the module is to develop students' knowledge of the principles and methods of evidence-based clinical practice so that they can apply those methods to assessing and treating communication disorders in children and adults. The learning outcomes of the module are expressed to students in the form of knowledge outcomes and skills outcomes. The intended knowledge outcomes are that students should be able to: (a) formulate answerable clinical questions; (b) search the literature for evidence-based research that addresses those questions; (c) assess the methodological quality of the research; and (d) apply the conclusions of evidence-based findings to clinical practice. The intended skills outcomes are that students should be able to: (a) develop information skills needed for EBP, including searching for relevant and high-quality literature using specialized bibliographic databases (e.g., Medline); (b) critically evaluate research evidence using the principles and methods of EBP; and (c) present a critical review of evidence relating to a specific area of clinical interest.

The final-year option modules at Newcastle are typically taught over a period of six weeks, with the EBP module meeting once a week for three hours. A short lecture is presented at the beginning of each class, followed by small group seminar discussions facilitated by each of the course instructors. Students are assigned a set of readings that they are to have read in advance of each week's class. The readings each week include one or more chapters from Greenhalgh (2006), which is the module's core text. This text presents the main elements of EBP in a readable format.[2] In addition, students read a set of research articles relating to intervention or assessment. These are updated each time the module is taught and are selected to reflect various study types (e.g., systematic reviews; randomized controlled trials, RCTs; diagnostic accuracy studies) and subject matter (e.g., stuttering, child language disorders, aphasia). The coverage is intentionally broad so that students are exposed to a wide range of clinical research across subdisciplines. Lectures typically focus on summarizing and elaborating general principles outlined in the textbook, while seminar discussions engage students in critically appraising research studies and drawing conclusions about their clinical practice. The following section briefly describes each of the weekly sessions.

The syllabus

Week 1. The first class begins with a brief lecture covering several topics. The first addresses the question: *What is evidence-based practice?* Several definitions, from a historical perspective and arising from EBP's origin in evidence-based medicine, are given as well as newer ones offered by Greenhalgh (2006) and Dollaghan (2007; see Table 1). This is followed by an introduction to how to construct answerable clinical questions using the standard PICO (patients, intervention, comparison group, outcomes) format and, having done that, how to search for high-quality evidence that addresses the question.

Students are then given a short written text about a young child who has been referred to an SLT as a result of failing a language screening. It represents the kind of information they might encounter in reading referral notes or a case history prior to conducting a clinical assessment. They then break up into small groups to discuss the text, identifying what they know and what they do not know about the information presented. This discussion requires 10–15 minutes when the students have had previous experience of case-based learning. The point of the exercise is to get students to discuss their knowledge of terminology (e.g., *screening*), assumptions made (e.g., about the accuracy of the screening), and the relation between factual statements and possible outcomes (e.g., whether there is an association between apparent risk factors and speech and language outcomes). Students are then asked to reflect on how they know what they know. This in turn leads to a discussion of different kinds of evidence, where to go to find it, and how to evaluate the quality of the evidence found.

This past year, we added a practical session to the course involving one of the University's medical librarians,[3] who

Table 1. Some definitions of evidence-based medicine and evidence-based practice

Definition	Source
"...the conscientious, explicit and judicious use of current best evidence in making decisions about the care of individual patients. The practice of evidence based medicine means integrating individual clinical expertise with the best available external clinical evidence from systematic research." (p. 71)	Sackett, Rosenberg, Gray, Haynes, and Richardson (1996)
"...the integration of the best research evidence with clinical expertise and patient values" (p. 1)	Sackett, Straus, Richardson, Rosenberg, and Haynes (2000)
"...the integration of the best research evidence with our clinical expertise and our patient's unique values and circumstances" (p. 1)	Straus, Richardson, Glasziou, and Haynes (2005)
"...the use of mathematical estimates of the risk of benefit and harm, derived from high-quality research on population samples, to inform clinical decision making in the diagnosis, investigation or management of individual patients." (p. 1)	Greenhalgh (2006)
"...the conscientious, explicit, and judicious integration of (1) best available *external* evidence from systematic research, (2) best available evidence *internal* to clinical practice, and (3) best available evidence concerning the preferences of a fully informed patient." (p. 2)	Dollaghan (2007)

demonstrated the use of specialist web-based research databases such as the Cochrane Library and Medline and how to search Medline using standard interfaces such as Ovid and PubMed. Students then worked through online exercises designed to give them first-hand experience of formulating PICO questions and using Medical Subject Headings (MeSH terms) to search for high-quality evidence.

Week 2.   The second class begins with a discussion of how different types of study design have been organized into hierarchies of evidence depending on the nature of the clinical question being asked (e.g., intervention, diagnosis) and illustrates one such hierarchy using the Oxford Centre for Evidence-Based Medicine's Levels of Evidence (Retrieved October 29, 2009, from http://www.cebm.net/index.aspx?o=1025). Students are then introduced to how the methodological quality of studies can be evaluated using critical appraisal checklists such as those compiled by the Scottish Intercollegiate Guidelines Network (SIGN; Retrieved October 29, 2009, from http:// www.sign.ac.uk/methodology/checklists.html). The lecture ends by introducing students to the first of several study designs: the randomized controlled trial (RCT). Students then break up into small groups to critically appraise one or more RCTs that they read in preparation for the seminar (e.g., Jones et al., 2005).

Week 3.   The third week focuses on critically evaluating evidence relating to clinical assessment (i.e., screening and diagnosis). The lecture illustrates some of the key concepts introduced in Chapter 7 of Greenhalgh (2006), which relate to how a clinical assessment (index test) can be validated against a reference standard. Key measures, such as test sensitivity, specificity,

and likelihood ratios are discussed using an example from the literature. Students are shown how to calculate such measures, and their confidence intervals, using the Stats Calculator on the Toronto Centre for Evidence-Based Medicine's website (Retrieved October 29, 2009, from http:// cebm.utoronto.ca/practise/ca/statscal/). From this, students are then shown how to determine the likelihood, or posttest probability, of a clinical condition using the nomogram on the Oxford CEBM's website (Retrieved October 29, 2009, from http://www.cebm. net/index.aspx?o=1161#). Reporting standards and critical appraisal checklists for diagnostic accuracy studies are also covered (see Klee, 2008). One or more diagnostic accuracy studies are then critically appraised by the students in the seminar that follows.

Week 4.   Systematic reviews and meta-analyses are discussed in this class, and, as is done each week, the relevant SIGN critical appraisal checklist is introduced for evaluating them. The seminar discussion that follows revolves around critically appraising one such systematic review (e.g., Law, Garrett, & Nye, 2004).

Week 5.   The topic of the penultimate class is applying EBP in clinical practice. One of the authors, a former manager of a large pediatric speech and language service within the National Health Service, speaks to the students of her experience of introducing and encouraging the use of EBP among practicing clinicians. Students are presented with clinical scenarios, which are then discussed.

Week 6.   Students are assessed during the final class meeting. Each student presents a 20-minute talk on a topic of their choosing, followed by 10 minutes of questions from the course instructors. To give students an idea of the kind of questions that could be asked,

Table 2. Examples given to students, in 2008–2009, for student presentations

Questions and rationale

(1) Does using sign language with normal-hearing babies and toddlers accelerate their language development?
  - Why ask this question? 'Baby Signs' programs are offered to parents of young children all over the world. The notice board in my GP's waiting room advertises such a group and at least one local SLT practice offers this as a form of intervention.
  - The claim on one website is that "Ten years of research have proved conclusively using Baby Signs not only leads to better communication; it also speeds up the process of learning to talk, stimulates intellectual development, enhances self esteem, and strengthens the bond between parent and infant."

(2) Is the Fast ForWord computer program an effective intervention in treating children with language impairment?
  - Why ask this question? The children I work with love computer games and this seems like an ideal way of getting them to attend to intervention tasks while having fun.

(3) How effective is the McGuire Program for treating adults who stammer?
  - Why ask this question? One of my clients asked me what I thought of this approach to intervention after reading what Gareth Gates had to say about it in the *Metro* newspaper.

Note. Not in PICO (patients, intervention, comparison group, outcomes) format.

the assessment brief contains examples of questions that might arise in clinical practice along with brief rationales (see Table 2). Students are asked to generate their own clinical question and include answers to the following in their presentations: (a) your question in PICO format and a brief rationale for why you are asking that question; (b) how you went about searching for evidence to answer your question (e.g., search engines and key words used); (c) how you decided which studies to include and exclude in your review; (d) list of the studies included in your review, summarized in a table based on the Cochrane reporting framework (7 columns: author + date, methods, participants, interventions, outcomes, notes, allocation concealment); (e) a critical appraisal of this evidence followed by your conclusion(s); and (f) suggestions for future research that would address your question. Each student submits a copy of their PowerPoint presentation, along with a list of references and the summary table outlined in (d) above.

The course website

In addition to lectures, seminar discussions and assigned readings, student learning is supported by electronic resources placed on Blackboard. The Blackboard website contains many EBP resources, including links to electronic databases (e.g., PubMed, National Library for Health, Cochrane Collaboration, Campbell Collaboration, What Works Clearinghouse, speechBITE). Blackboard also contains links to recent studies in communication disorders arranged by subject area and by study design (e.g., systematic reviews, RCTs, case-control studies, cohort studies, single case designs), copies of lecture notes and handouts, links to reporting standards and critical appraisal checklists, evidence-based medicine (EBM) websites, and other resources.

The success of the EBP module is in part dependent on the groundwork laid by other staff prior to students enrolling in this module. As indicated earlier, students at Newcastle take modules in research methods in each of their first three years and so arrive in the EBP module with a foundation in research design and statistics. They also have completed most of their formal coursework and clinical placements and are well on the way to completing their undergraduate dissertations. That said, if there is one criticism of the EBP module, it is that many students have told us that they wished the module had been offered earlier in their degree program and that it should be compulsory. The next step, then, in introducing EBP into the curriculum at Newcastle involved changing a clinic placement in the third year of the program, and this is described next.

THE UNDERGRADUATE EBP CLINICAL PLACEMENT

The motivation for the more explicit inclusion of EBP principles into clinical placements on the undergraduate program came from three sources: the use of case-based problem solving (CBPS) as a method of curriculum delivery, the outcome of training in the principles of EBP for those Clinical Educators, and the collaborative relationship between the University and practicing SLTs in the region.

Since 1999, a substantial amount of the learning and teaching on the pre-registration SLT degree programs at Newcastle has been in the form of CBPS (Whitworth et al., 2004). Students are required to read and evaluate literature related to a clinical case presented in class and, in small groups, develop a management plan over the course of several weeks. The critical use of the evidence base is therefore integral to this form of curriculum delivery. However, it became apparent that this was implicit, rather than explicit, and students did not view these as transferable skills to use as part of the EBP palette, but narrowly applied them within the CBPS modules. This observation is supported by the fact that when EBP principles and skills were explicitly taught in the final year EBP module of the undergraduate program, they were often greeted as novel.

One of the authors provides training in the principles of EBP to practicing SLTs through a regional research Special Interest Group.

A common complaint from SLTs is that the working week does not allow adequate time for the formulation of questions about their practice and the subsequent investigation and analysis to answer those questions, despite the obvious benefits to clients. Some SLTs already required students on placement to investigate literature related to their clients and to evaluate the available evidence; this was clearly a resource that could be tapped further. In addition, there is no repository of previously asked questions, and SLTs were aware that they could be replicating work that had already been done by a colleague in a neighboring service. The need to share questions and outcomes was identified as a priority in the clinical community.

In the United Kingdom, as in most countries where pre-registration training for SLTs is regulated by a professional or statutory body, there are a minimum number of hours of clinical practice required of students. There is a requirement for these to be in a variety of settings and to cover a broad range of client groups. At Newcastle, the first two placements for undergraduate students take place in the campus clinics where students deliver interventions to clients with acquired or developmental speech, language, and/or literacy disorders. Subsequent placements take place outside the University across the North East of England with locally employed SLTs serving as Clinical Educators. The University has developed and nurtured a close working relationship with SLT services in the National Health Service and local authorities across the North East. In addition to personal contacts between university staff and individual SLTs, there is a wide range of professional activities that include the following: supporting Special Interest Groups; research collaborations including specialist clinicians as teachers and examiners on the degree programs; being responsive to the needs of the services in a professional context; and regular meetings to plan and to oversee student placements. Some of the students' assignments are designed to be of direct benefit to the SLT and their service. For example, the first of two final-year undergraduate placements involves the student undertaking a piece of work for the SLT, such as an audit, a small-scale service evaluation, or the development of therapy materials. It is clear that they are not research projects but they may be precursors to pilot research projects. Some of these have led to publications and external funding. It is in this context of collaboration that EBP was integrated into the third-year undergraduate clinical placement.

In the second semester of the third year, undergraduate students have a 6-week full-time block placement, which is partially assessed through a 3,000-word written case report about a selected client. In the 2007–2008 academic year the EBP element was added to this assessment in the form of an investigation of a PICO question related to the client or client group concerned, the results of which were to be presented in an appendix to the case report. The appendices would then be made available to SLTs in the region through the University's secure SLT extranet.

Clinical Educators who were to supervise students on the first placement were introduced to the principles of EBP and requirements of the placement in a half-day workshop. The workshop covered how to formulate a PICO question relating to an aspect of the intervention process, levels of evidence, and the use of critical appraisal checklists. The role of Clinical Educators was to guide the students so that questions were appropriate and also fulfilled the needs of the SLT. Preparation for students took place during induction week at the beginning of the academic year. This was planned to give students opportunity to practice critical appraisal during the CBPS modules in the first semester. The students were given a half-day workshop introducing the principles of EBP and levels of evidence, a recap on searching for evidence (which they were all familiar with from library skills training), and evaluation of the literature using a simple critical appraisal checklist (Bury & Mead, 1998). At this stage the more detailed and specific checklists such as SIGN (Retrieved October 29, 2009, from http://www.sign.ac.uk) or CASP (Retrieved October 29, 2009, from http://www.phru.nhs.uk/Pages/PHD/CASP.htm) were not used because there was no opportunity for staff to check that the students had chosen the correct checklist for the type of paper they were appraising. The relationship between the EBP section and the case report was made explicit, so that the intrinsic value of investigating the evidence was clear to students. During the workshop they practiced critical appraisal in small groups of 3–4 students on a paper that had been read before class; then, as a class group, they reflected on the difference between reading a paper and critically appraising a paper. Integrating knowledge from modules such as Research Methods with theoretical and clinical knowledge, the students were able to accurately and fairly appraise literature within that session. During the reflective discussion they commented on how the critical appraisal process and the checklist supported them to question material they would have previously taken at face value.

A standard method of recording the outcome of the question was devised to enable students and clinicians to easily access the outcomes and update them in the future. The students were asked to record the following: (a) question (in PICO format); (b) keywords used and databases searched; (c) relevant papers found and rationale for choosing and rejecting papers; (d) summary of relevant findings and level of evidence; (e) statement of findings (i.e., the answer to the question).

This has resulted in a web resource for the North East SLT community of nearly 60 EBP questions to date. The topics chosen are diverse, reflecting the focus of the students' clinical placements and the range of client groups that SLTs work with, as seen in the examples below:

- Is the use of an oral communication approach (no sign language used) more beneficial than a total communication approach (sign and spoken language used) in the development of speech and language in adolescents with hearing impairments?

- Is narrative therapy an effective intervention for young children with specific language impairment/language delay for improving the quality of their oral narratives and performance in the classroom?

- In school age children with developmental delay unable to meet their communication needs through natural speech, using therapist delivered augmentative and alternative communication (AAC) intervention, are aided or unaided forms of AAC best to improve functional communication?

- In people with aphasia who have marked verb impairment, should verbs be treated within sentences or as single words to achieve the greatest generalization to functional use?

THE MSC IN EVIDENCE-BASED PRACTICE IN COMMUNICATION DISORDERS

As we stated earlier, Speech and language therapists in the United Kingdom are expected to deliver evidence-based treatment and experience problems in doing so. Taken seriously, doing evidence-based practice means that every clinical choice should be based on the best available evidence. In practice there are a number of obstacles that

any practitioner faces. First, any clinician makes many clinical decisions every day, facing questions such as: (a) What is the best way to assess this client? (b) Given their assessment results, what conclusions can be drawn about the nature of their underlying disorder(s)? (c) Given a conclusion about the underlying disorder(s), what approach to treatment is likely to be most effective? and (d) Is there evidence on how it is best to deliver the therapy?

Managers of services are usually working with limited resources when compared to the potential demand and have to make decisions about the prioritization of services and how they can be most effectively and economically delivered. The questions that clinicians and managers face are subtly different. The clinician is faced with decisions about an individual client, whereas the manager has to make much broader strategic decisions about the allocation of resources to client groups (that is, populations).

Second, there is the problem of time; many of the clinician's decisions have to be made "on the fly" during a face-to-face session with a client (O'Connor & Pettigrew, 2009; Zipoli & Kennedy, 2005). There is often little time to investigate the existing evidence from the literature and develop a proper evidence-based decision. Perhaps as a result, some clinicians may revert to established customs of clinical practice, while being uncomfortably aware that these may not be based on good evidence (but usually unsure whether that is the case). Moreover, decisions about the treatment or assessment of any individual client are very specific. The question might be, for this client with this particular profile of strengths and weaknesses, is there evidence that one particular treatment might be more effective than another? It could be argued that restricting the available assessments and treatments to those that can be justified on the basis of a critical appraisal of the evidence would free the time necessary for further evaluations; unfortunately there is no evidence that this is the case.

The third problem is how to access the available evidence. Clinicians often, with justification, point out that much of the available evidence can be hard to retrieve, and their employers may not be able to give them access to all of the relevant journals. This is probably a problem that is more acute for SLTs than for doctors; given decisions about journal subscriptions, employers often (reasonably) consider speech pathology-oriented journals a minority interest.

Fourth, clinicians and managers have to think about how to assess—how to weight—the available evidence. Speech and language pathology is a field where, for good reasons (Hegde, 2007) there is rarely relevant evidence from well-conducted RCTs. And, it has been argued, RCTs do not necessarily yield the best evidence for making decisions about individual clients drawn from heterogeneous populations (Hegde, 2007; Howard, 1986; Pring, 2004). Practitioners are then faced with complex decisions in evaluating the evidence from other sources of evidence such as small group designs and single-subject experimental designs (SSEDs; but see the special issue of *Evidence-Based Communication Assessment and Intervention* on meta-analysis of SSEDs; Schlosser & Sigafoos, 2008). While there are clear and well-accepted methods for combining RCTs into a meta-analysis, it is still very unclear how one might combine or weight other sources of evidence.[4] All the evidence needs to be assessed and weighed: as Guyatt et al. (2000) pointed out, "any statement to the effect that there is no evidence addressing the effect of a particular treatment is a non sequitur. The evidence may be extremely weak—the unsystematic observation of a single clinician, or generalization from only indirectly related physiologic studies—but there is always evidence" (p. 1293).

Service managers will be making decisions prioritizing services across a population, with a view to both the relative costs and the size of the benefits to the client groups. Here, RCTs that document the mean change from an intervention across a population are more relevant. But there are problems: RCTs for the relevant population often do not exist. When they do, the populations from which the clients are drawn may not be strictly comparable to the client group the manager is considering. The question then is how to weight such evidence. When they do not, clinicians will have to rely on other sources of evidence (e.g., SSEDs, small-group studies).

The other issue in weighting evidence is methodological quality. Does a study, of whatever kind, yield convincing evidence that supports the conclusions? While existing checklists can be helpful, assessing this with any reliability requires skills in understanding both experimental design and statistics. Critical evaluation at this level requires skills in a domain where few clinicians feel confident.

These constitute serious practical problems for any clinician or service manager trying to meet their responsibility to deliver services that are evidence based. One option—and probably one that is widely adopted—is to rely on practice guidelines that are (or claim to be) evidence based in making decisions. Such practice guidelines are widely available and are produced by a number of different professional organizations and other sources. There are also systematic reviews of the evidence on particular issues published in various journals (including this one). The problem in following such guidelines is that, although they may all claim to be evidence based, they do not necessarily reach the same conclusions. This is often because they place different amounts of weight on different sources of evidence. Cochrane reviews, for example, can only consider RCTs as evidence; in contrast, for example, Cicerone et al. (2000, 2005) in their review for the American Congress of Rehabilitation Medicine are willing to entertain a much wider range of evidence including case series and single case studies.

The effect of contradictory or inconsistent guidelines means that the individual clinician or manager needs to come to a view of how well founded the guidelines are in relation to their individual decisions. The result is that, even with evidence-based guidelines, clinicians need the skills of critical appraisal to be able to deliver evidence-based practice.

Our experience of delivering training in EBP to practicing clinicians is that it tends to expose their lack of expertise in the domains necessary for assembling and evaluating the evidence. A one- or two-day course does little more than reinforce the participants' view of the difficulty of really doing EBP. This is not surprising, because, as we have argued, there are real and substantial problems in implementing the approach.

The program

In September 2009, we started an MSc in Evidence-Based Practice in Communication Disorders at Newcastle University. The aims are to provide clinicians and managers with the skills needed to implement evidence-based treatment and assessment in their clinical practice.

The skills we will seek to develop are those needed to address (some of) the problems[5] we have just described, but also, simply, the skills needed for EBP: (a) understanding how to pose questions that are both answerable and address questions in clinical practice; (b) the ability to search systematically for all of the relevant evidence; (c) the skills needed to evaluate critically the existing evidence, using all the relevant sources. This depends on critical knowledge of research methods and statistics. This is

essential for moving on from relatively primitive check-list-based evaluations of evidence so that students can bring more penetrating and critical understanding to the evidence available.

The point is made to our students that if we depended only on evaluation of pre-existing therapies and assessments there would be stagnation. British Master's courses almost always require a research component; in Newcastle's new MSc, this involves training in research methods and, in addition, conducting a research project that evaluates an assessment or a therapy method. This involves developing many relevant research skills, which, beyond the theoretical skills in experimental design and analysis, involve more practical/administrative issues such as confronting ethical approval procedures, identifying appropriate statistical support (where necessary), and participant recruitment and consent. This confrontation with the practicalities of empirical research will also inform evaluation of others' research.

EBP can encourage a rather rigid approach to the evaluation of evidence, with unblinking adherence to some received "hierarchy of evidence" (which is often reinforced by using checklists). Recognizing that different kinds of evidence have different impacts on different issues, we hope to develop in students a more sophisticated appreciation of the strengths and weaknesses of different sources of evidence that should inform a critical synthesis of the evidence on any specific issue. This is done, in part, by helping students gain an appreciation for the wide-range of research designs employed (e.g., RCTs, cohort studies, case-control studies, SSEDs, diagnostic accuracy studies) and the ways in which these can be critically appraised.

We are aware that for a course to have any impact on the use of EBP in speech–language pathology it has to be accessible to clinicians and managers who are in full-time posts. To make appropriate study leave more feasible, the program is delivered as a set of six very intensive three-day modules with the expectation that students carry out a great deal of independent work in the periods in between. The first cohort of students has just begun the MSc program, and we look forward both to their progress and to reporting on how the program evolves in the years ahead.

ACKNOWLEDGMENTS

We gratefully acknowledge the students who enrolled in the EBP module at Newcastle in the first four years it was offered. Their enthusiasm for learning about and applying the methods of EBP to explore clinical questions bodes well for the next generation of professionals and the people they serve.

Declaration of interest: The authors were employed by Newcastle University during the time the curriculum developments discussed in this paper were implemented, and they alone are responsible for the content and writing of this paper.

NOTES

1. The book's title, *Bad Science*, is also the name of the author's column that appears each Saturday in *The Guardian* newspaper and on the web (http://www.guardian.co.uk/science/series/badscience).
2. Students have been uniformly positive about Greenhalgh's book, and because of that we continue to use it as the main course text. Since we began offering the course, Dollaghan's (2007) discipline-specific introduction to EBP in communication disorders has appeared, and we include it on the syllabus as a supplemental reading. We also suggest several other resources (e.g., Ajetunmobi, 2002; Haynes, Sackett, Guyatt, & Tugwell, 2006; Straus, Richardson, Glasziou, & Haynes, 2005) for future reference or for students wanting more advanced discussion of topics in Greenhalgh's book. In addition, students are made aware of resources such as the journal, *Evidence-Based Communication Assessment and Intervention*.
3. In the second and third years of the undergraduate program, students receive practical tutorials on the use of more general search tools such as the Web of Science, Scopus, and Google Scholar from the Speech and Language Sciences liaison librarian.
4. We are not aware of any consensus for how information from well-conducted experimental group designs could be combined with information from well-conducted SSEDs. More problematic is how evidence from different kinds of studies (e.g., RCTs, small-group cross-over designs, SSEDs) could be combined into a single meta-analysis. Combining studies of different designs requires the evaluator to make a number of assumptions, many of which cannot easily be justified. Arguably, the weight that should be given to different kinds of studies varies depending on the issues addressed, and there is as yet no consensus on how this should be done.
5. There are some problems an educational course cannot address. The most obvious are lack of time and access to the relevant literature. Clinicians and managers, if they are enjoined to deliver EBP, necessarily require the time to assess the available evidence and access to the necessary sources. Those are employers' responsibilities.

REFERENCES

Ajetunmobi, O. (2002). *Making sense of critical appraisal.* London: Hodder Arnold.

Bury, T., & Mead, J. (1998). *Evidence based healthcare: A practical guide for therapists.* London: Butterworth-Heinemann.

Cicerone, K. D., Dahlberg, C., Kalmar, K., Langenbahn, D. M., Malec, J. F., Bergquist, T. F., et al. (2000). Evidence-based cognitive rehabilitation: Recommendations for clinical practice. *Archives of Physical Medicine and Rehabilitation, 81,* 1596–1615.

Cicerone, K. D., Dahlberg, C., Malec, J. F., Langenbahn, D. M., Felicetti, T., Kneipp, S., et al. (2005). Evidence-based cognitive rehabilitation: Updated review of the literature from 1998 through 2002. *Archives of Physical Medicine and Rehabilitation, 86,* 1681–1692.

Dollaghan, C. A. (2007). *The handbook for evidence-based practice in communication disorders.* Baltimore, MD: Paul H. Brookes Publishing Co.

Goldacre, B. (2008). *Bad science.* London: Fourth Estate.

Greenhalgh, T. (2001). *How to read a paper: The basics of evidence-based medicine* (2nd ed.). London: BMJ Books.

Greenhalgh, T. (2006). *How to read a paper: The basics of evidence-based medicine* (3rd ed.). Oxford, UK: Blackwell.

Guyatt, G. H., Haynes, R. B., Jaeschke, R. Z., Cook, D. J., Green, L., Naylor, C. D., et al. (2000). Users' guides to the medical literature: XXV. Evidence-based medicine: principles for applying the users' guides to patient care. *Journal of the American Medical Association, 284,* 1290–1296.

Haynes, R. B., Sackett, D. L., Guyatt, G. H., & Tugwell, P. (2006). *Clinical epidemiology: How to do clinical practice research* (3rd ed.). Philadelphia: Lippincott Williams & Wilkins.

Health Professions Council. (2007). *Standards of proficiency—speech and language therapists*. Retrieved October 29, 2009, from http://www.hpc-uk.org/assets/documents/10000529Standards_of_Proficiency_SLTs.pdf

Hegde, M. N. (2007). A methodological review of randomized clinical trials. *Communicative Disorders Review, 1,* 17–38.

Howard, D. (1986). Beyond randomised controlled trials: The case for effective case studies of the effects of treatment in aphasia. *British Journal of Disorders of Communication, 21,* 89–102.

Jones, M., Onslow, M., Packman, A., Williams, S., Ormond, T., Schwarz, I., et al. (2005). Randomised controlled trial of the Lidcombe programme of early stuttering intervention. *British Medical Journal, 331,* 659–663.

Klee, T. (2008). Considerations for appraising diagnostic studies of communication disorders. *Evidence-Based Communication Assessment and Intervention, 2,* 1–12.

Law, J., Garrett, Z., & Nye, C. (2004). The efficacy of treatment for children with developmental speech and language delay/disorder: A meta-analysis. *Journal of Speech, Language, and Hearing Research, 47,* 924–943.

O'Connor, S., & Pettigrew, C. M. (2009). The barriers perceived to prevent the successful implementation of evidence-based practice by speech and language therapists. *International Journal of Language & Communication Disorders, 44,* 1018–1035.

Pring, T. (2004). Ask a silly question: Two decades of troublesome trials. *International Journal of Language & Communication Disorders, 39,* 285–302.

Sackett, D. L., Rosenberg, W. M. C., Gray, J. A. M., Haynes, R. B., & Richardson, W. S. (1996). Evidence based medicine: What it is and what it isn't. *British Medical Journal, 312,* 71–72.

Sackett, D. L., Straus, S. E., Richardson, W. S., Rosenberg, W., & Haynes, R. B. (2000). *Evidence-based medicine: How to practice and teach EBM* (2nd ed.). Edinburgh, UK: Churchill Livingstone.

Schlosser, R. W., & Sigafoos, J. (2008). Meta-analysis of single-subject experimental designs: Why now? *Evidence-Based Communication Assessment and Intervention, 2,* 117–119.

Straus, S. E., Richardson, W. S., Glasziou, P., & Haynes, R. B. (2005). *Evidence-based medicine: How to practice and teach EBM* (3rd ed.). Edinburgh, UK: Elsevier Churchill Livingstone.

Whitworth, A., Franklin, S., & Dodd, B. (2004). Case-based problem solving for speech and language therapy students. In S. Brumfitt (Ed.), *Innovations in professional education for speech and language therapists* (pp. 29–50). London: Whurr.

Zipoli Jr., R. P., & Kennedy, M. (2005). Evidence-based practice among speech-language pathologists: Attitudes, utilization, and barriers. *American Journal of Speech-Language Pathology, 14,* 208–220.

Evidence-based Communication Assessment and Intervention
2009, 3(4), 208–219

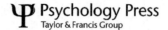

Ψ Psychology Press
Taylor & Francis Group

Case-based learning: One route to evidence-based practice

Patricia McCabe, Alison Purcell, Elise Baker*, Catherine Madill*, & David Trembath*

Discipline of Speech Pathology, The University of Sydney, Sydney, Australia

Abstract

Discussion about the use of evidence-based practice (EBP) by speech pathologists is widespread yet little is known on how to teach EBP to student speech pathologists. This paper illustrates how a case-based approach to learning and teaching (CBL) has been used to facilitate undergraduate and master's level students' understanding and conduct of EBP across the speech pathology curriculum at the University of Sydney. A definition of CBL is provided followed by an overview of how students learn to manage cases within a framework, known as the Client Management Process (CMP). The CMP was designed to guide students' evidence-based clinical reasoning and decision making across the stages of contact with clients, from referral to dismissal. Preliminary evaluation and comments by both students and instructors on the value and difficulties associated with using a CBL to teach EBP are presented.

Keywords: *Case based learning; Evidence based practice; Speech language pathology; Curriculum; Constructive alignment.*

"All cases are unique and very similar to others."

    T. S. Eliot (1950)

Evidence-based practice (EBP) poses two significant challenges for instructors involved in university speech pathology programs. One is to facilitate students' learning of the fundamentals of EBP such as searching for and evaluating the literature, and the second is to facilitate students' development of clinical expertise, so that graduate clinicians can integrate the ideals afforded by published research with the complexities and constraints of real life, in their day-to-day decision making. The purpose of this paper is to illustrate how a case-based approach to learning and teaching (CBL) has been used to facilitate students' understanding and conduct of EBP across the speech pathology curriculum at the University of Sydney and thus to address these two challenges.

Instructors in university speech pathology programs have traditionally thought themselves the literature skills required to conduct EBP—that is, to form a question and to search and evaluate the literature to reach conclusions about the best available evidence. Although research has shown that universities succeed in imparting literature-based skills to their allied health graduates (Pain, Magill-Evans, Darrah, Hagler, & Warren, 2004), research examining allied health professionals' barriers to conducting EBP suggests that they are not confident evaluating the quality of research nor understanding the statistical analyses reported in research papers (e.g., Metcalfe et al., 2001). Clinicians also believe that the implications for clinical practice are not clearly reported in published

*All equal third author.

For correspondence: Patricia McCabe, Discipline of Speech Pathology, Faculty of Health Sciences, The University of Sydney, PO Box 170 Lidcombe NSW 1825, Australia. E-mail: p.mccabe@usyd.edu.au

Source of funding: No source of funding reported.

http://www.psypress.com/EBCAI

DOI: 10.1080/17489530903399145

research (O'Connor & Pettigrew, 2009), suggesting that even when clinicians can search for and understand the evidence, the challenge remains knowing how to integrate published evidence with clinical expertise and client values and preferences on a daily basis (Pennington et al., 2005). The existence of such barriers means that EBP "has not become a regular part of clinical practice" (Brackenbury, Burroughs, & Hewitt, 2008, p. 78). There would seem to be a divide between research evidence and clinical practice that speech pathologists find difficult to bridge.

While there are a number of possible strategies and frameworks for guiding speech pathologists' application of research evidence to clinical practice in the workplace (e.g., Gillam & Gillam, 2006), it is harder to find higher education literature which suggests how this divide might feasibly be addressed in university programs. Academic programs need to establish ways in which the real-life application of evidence can be taught in a way that both facilitates theoretical learning and ensures skills transfer to the workplace.

Some authors have suggested that learning how to apply evidence to clinical scenarios is best achieved in a clinical education setting (Gillam & Gillam, 2008; Goldstein, 2008). This raises two issues. First, clinical educators are drawn from the speech pathology population in general, and it would seem that these clinicians, regardless of experience or place of employment, are also having difficulty applying the evidence to their clinical practice (Togher et al., 2009). Secondly, such a practice perpetuates the research evidence–clinical practice divide in the mind of the students, reinforcing the lack of applicability outside the classroom of what is taught inside it.

PROBLEM-BASED LEARNING

Problem-based learning (PBL) has been suggested as an alternate approach for bridging the divide between research and practice, and as such facilitating students' conduct of EBP. While PBL has shown promise in this regard in the fields of medicine and nursing (Fineout-Overton, Stillwell, & Kent, 2008), PBL would seem to be out of reach financially for many speech pathology programs, as it requires relatively higher resource levels than didactic teaching (Finucane, Shannon, & McGrath, 2009).

CASE-BASED LEARNING

An alternate solution to this dilemma is case-based learning (CBL). CBL represents middle ground between PBL and traditional pedagogy and starts with the adult learning premises that adults learn best when what is to be learned is both meaningful to the individual and relates to real life (Knowles, Holton, & Swanson, 2005). Real cases facilitate learning of clinical and theoretical material and presumably facilitate the application of research evidence to clinical practice.

A few different definitions of CBL exist in the literature. For example, Rybarczyk, Baines, McVey, Thompson, and Wilkins (2007) define CBL as a "method that uses case studies as active learning tools" (p. 181). For the purpose of this paper, CBL means the use of real-life or hypothetical clinical cases to promote student thinking and learning in ways that simulate clinical practice. CBL learning activities encourage clinical problem solving and reasoning activities in individuals and groups and contrast with the didactic delivery of case-based information or clinical vignettes by instructors to students.

Traditional didactic teaching with case examples typically involves the presentation of small portions of clinical information, which are used to illustrate a theoretical point. Subjects taught in this manner typically present many cases in one semester, few of which meet the criteria for a CBL case. To illustrate this point, in a traditionally taught voice subject at the University of Sydney, there were 35 different clinical snapshots to illustrate each of the major diagnostic or therapeutic issues. In the CBL curriculum there are only 5 cases, which, when used across the semester, allow the students to discover the principles of voice assessment and intervention. The 5 CBL cases being rich, detailed, revisited, and complex are remembered in clinical practice; while the 35 case snippets may be forgotten.

One advantage of CBL is that it allows for competency development in clinical reasoning in the classroom setting, thus conserving the critical resource of clinical placements (Lincoln & McCabe, 2005). Further, the use of real cases means that when students are exposed to individual patients in clinical settings their classroom-based learning is reactivated and facilitates integration with learning in the new setting, thus crossing the hypothesized research–practice gap. CBL capitalizes on the idea that "students learn what they care about and remember what they understand" (Ericksen, 1984, p. 51).

What is a case?

A case is the real, detailed information about a client presented over time. The case can be individuals, groups, classes, or organizations but more than one piece of information needs to be included. In a systematic review of what makes a case effective, Kim and colleagues (2006) suggest that five features are essential. The case must be relevant, realistic, engaging, challenging, and instructional.

To be relevant, cases need to be at a sufficient level of complexity, to be presented in a narrative manner, and address the student learning objectives. Realistic cases are ones that are presented to students with irrelevant information left in so that the richness and complexity of people's lives

are maintained. This real-life messiness both adds to the authenticity of the case and ensures that the students are engaged with and remember the case. Such distractor information teaches students to sort clinical data for relevance. At this point it is worth remembering that EBP requires clinicians to understand clients in all their complexity and to take this complexity into account in their clinical decision making.

How are cases used in a CBL framework?

CBL requires that the students interact with the case in a meaningful way. Students are required to engage with cases via learning activities to understand the theoretical and practical considerations of the materials being presented. More specifically, cases are used to introduce students to new ideas, to identify the most important pieces of information, to generate hypotheses, to develop appropriate assessment and management plans, and to facilitate reflection on management of the case.

Time is an important factor in using CBL. Cases recur within the curriculum as students learn to manage the complexity of clinical practice. Recurrence may be within a subject or across subjects. Individual cases are shared with students over time so that the different presentations of a given disorder can be explored. Thus in stuttering, seeing how the disorder presents in a 3-year-old is insufficient to understand the various clinical paths that a client who stutters may take over time. Instead of presenting a series of different children as snapshots in time, a case-based approach follows one child over time.

A CASE EXAMPLE: CBL AT THE UNIVERSITY OF SYDNEY

At the University of Sydney we have adopted CBL in both our undergraduate and master's level speech pathology professional preparation courses. We use a range of approaches to the development and use of cases across the curriculum with a guiding set of principles that were collectively developed across the whole teaching team. Using CBL has allowed us to reduce the silo nature of teaching in individual subjects through the use of cases across academic subjects and the integration of multiple areas of academic content into single, more complex cases.

In some subjects one case runs the whole semester, with students exploring the various curriculum issues through the lens of one client presented as a series of consultations over time. Other subjects have a small set of cases that exemplify the diversity and complexity of speech pathology practice. For example, in the Voice Sciences and Disorders subjects, five cases are used to explicitly teach the conceptual framework of EBP in voice, with each case being represented through topics of referral, assessment, diagnosis, intervention, and discharge. One of these voice cases is a child with a phonological impairment (presented in a previous subject) who subsequently developed vocal nodules. As the cases are introduced, reviewed, or extended, concepts and skills relevant to the conduct of EBP are explicitly taught.

Case management process

In order to introduce students to cases in a systematic and EBP manner, a Client Management Process (CMP) framework was developed. The CMP is a framework that guides students' critical thinking as they consider how to make day-to-day evidence-based clinical decisions from the point of client referral to dismissal. The CMP framework builds on and extends the steps discussed in the literature about evidence-based decision making. Traditionally, the steps for engaging in EBP have been described as (a) generating a specific clinical question,

(b) searching for relevant published literature, (c) critically evaluating the literature, (d) applying the evidence, and (e) evaluating and monitoring the outcome (e.g., Sackett et al., 1996). Across this literature, discussions about the steps for engaging in EBP have typically focused on treatment or intervention-related decisions. We saw a need for students to consider the conventional steps of EBP (question→searching→ critiquing→applying→evaluating) at each stage in the management of a case.

Thus, our CMP involves four broad stages:

(1) Gathering information about the presenting problem for the case.

(2) Determining a preliminary diagnosis.

(3) Planning, implementing, and analyzing the results of an evidence-based assessment.

(4) Developing an appropriate management plan, which may include the selection of an evidence-based intervention approach in light of the information gathered from Stages 1 through 3.

At each of these stages, students use the steps for engaging in EBP, so as to make clinical decisions reflecting the best possible care for each case. Cases are typically presented as series of consultations, representing the process that is typical of speech pathologists working with clients and their families. This involves starting with a referral and moving through assessment, intervention, review, and potentially discharge. At each stage, students are required to generate relevant to their cases and an EBP approach to management. General questions might include: What are the characteristics of children with speech sound disorders? In what ways are the presenting characteristics of the case similar or different to the children in published literature? What is the best way to accurately diagnose specific language impairment in 4-year-old children? Do we know what the case's explicit preferences might be? Specific PICO questions about assessment, diagnosis and intervention are developed following discussion of the literature on the general questions. At each stage, the students are encouraged to find, review, critically appraise, and reflect on the evidence in published literature and to work in collaboration with peers and their instructor to generate evidence-based solutions to the questions. In doing so, the cases provide an engaging framework in which students learn to implement EBP.

Each stage of the CMP is also linked to the Speech Pathology Australia's Competency Based Occupational Standards for beginning-level speech pathologists (Speech Pathology Australia, 2001). These competencies are the minimum skills, knowledge, and attitudes required to enter the speech pathology profession in Australia and are divided into seven units of competency including assessment, assessment analysis and interpretation, planning speech pathology intervention, and speech pathology intervention.

Students engage with the cases both during their classes and asynchronously via a secure online platform. This resource includes accessing the case-specific file, and audio and video content from an online case resource system and online discussion of case materials. These activities support the in-class discussion and other learning tasks.

Examples of learning and teaching using a CBL framework

Speech sound disorders: Teaching in the undergraduate program. In the first year of the undergraduate speech pathology program students undertake a subject in speech sound disorders prior to commencing their clinical experience in their second year. In this subject students are invited to assume the role of a beginning clinician working with three other speech pathologists (class peers) in a Community Health setting. Consented de-identified file content is made available to the students in a graduated manner in conjunction with relevant video samples of assessment and intervention sessions. Students begin considering the nature of the problem and generate solutions for the ongoing management of the case. The structure of the academic subject mirrors the stages of professional contact that a speech pathologist might have with a child and their family for management of unintelligible speech. Following the initial referral, the students gather information from multiple perspectives about the nature of the problem, Stage 1 of the CMP. These perspectives typically include the research literature, views from parents, teachers, and the child himself, and the opinions of experts as expressed in textbooks and other resources. Having explored a series of questions and answers about the presenting problem, the students engage in Stage 2—generating a preliminary diagnosis. The students then engage in Stage 3 and generate an evidence-based assessment plan. At this point specific clinical questions are generated and answered via critical evaluation of the literature. For example, for a preschool child with unintelligible speech, is a single-word sample from a published test as valid and reliable as a 10-minute conversational speech sample for diagnosing a speech sound disorder? For a preschool child with unintelligible speech, is a computer-based phonological analysis as accurate as a manual independent and relational phonological analysis? As part of Stage 3, the students analyze actual assessment data for the case gathered by the instructor. The students also learn how to complete an in-depth independent and relational phonological analysis. Having completed the analysis, the students then complete Stage 4 of the CMP. At this point they engage in the more traditional steps associated with EBP, generating general background questions followed by a PICO question—for example: (a) General background question: What interventions are described in the literature for children with speech sound disorders?, (b) PICO question: Which intervention, (I), minimal pairs or multiple oppositions (C), is the most successful for improving intelligibility (O) in a preschool-aged child with a severe phonological impairment (P)?—and searching for and evaluating published intervention research.

As the subject progresses, four other cases of varying complexity are introduced. The additional cases contrast with the initial case to facilitate the transfer of knowledge to other clinical scenarios. In the latter weeks of the semester, families who have a child with a speech impairment visit the class to discuss their experience of raising a child who has unintelligible speech and share their insights on the experience of working with speech pathologists. This visit helps to highlight how client values and preferences might be integrated with clinical service factors and published research evidence in the management of speech sound disorders in children.

Lifelong disability. For many students, learning to work with individuals with lifelong disability is a new and confronting experience. The use of CBL allows students to work through a series of real, challenging cases in a safe and systematic way. Cases in this subject feature children and adolescents with physical and intellectual disability. In addition to the standard file-based information, video footage of clinicians working with the individuals and their families and recordings of interviews involving caregivers and a member of the university staff are included in the cases. Cases in this subject

have been developed in collaboration with the individuals featured in the cases, their families, and the professionals providing services at that time.

In a case involving a preschool-aged child with cerebral palsy, for example, students recommend an appropriate augmentative and alternative communication (AAC) system based on their review of the research literature, information contained in reports and file notes, and the views of the child's mother as expressed during the recorded interview. The real-life impact of clinician's decisions and expertise on the clients and their families is apparent in these supporting materials. Further, the presentation of file notes, individualized educational plans, and interview recordings, enables students to consider the impact of the preferences of the clients and families on the decision-making process. Through this process, students have the opportunity to form a deeply integrated view of their future professional role and the principles of EBP in a supported and structured learning environment.

Hearing impairment, craniofacial anomalies, and cultural and linguistic diversity. In the CBL curriculum a single subject using one case was developed to provide speech pathology students with knowledge on hearing impairment, hearing devices, craniofacial anomalies, and cultural and linguistic diversity. This information had previously been taught across five subjects over 110 hours of traditional teaching.

Students work with a single case over six consultations. The first consultation introduces them to the case, a three-week-old infant from a minority cultural background who presents to the Intake Clinic of a tertiary hospital with possible feeding difficulties and a "double refer" result on her infant hearing screening. Students meet this client over a further five visits or consultations from age 3 months to 10 years, 6 months. At each consultation students must grapple with a new diagnosis and use EBP to select the most appropriate methods of assessment and intervention for the client. For instance, at the second consultation the client has a diagnosis of a moderate sensorineural hearing loss, at the third consultation conductive hearing loss is present, at the fourth consultation a diagnosis of submucous cleft palate is revealed, at the fifth consultation the client's hearing levels have deteriorated to a profound sensorineural loss, and in the final consultation the client's speech is impacted by changes in dentition.

Speech sound disorders: Teaching in the master's program.   The above three examples demonstrate the use of the CMP in large- and small-group teaching from beginner through to advanced-level students. This approach is the most common CBL framework used across the curriculum but the flexibility of CBL allows for other approaches as appropriate.

An example of an alternate approach is to include a live case in a demonstration clinic in which the instructor assesses and treats an individual pediatric client with complex phonological issues. For our beginning master's students, who have had neither face-to-face experience nor substantial observation of speech pathology practice, academic classes are interwoven with the demonstration clinic. In the weekly class preceding the demonstration clinic, students are asked to explore issues of EBP in anticipation of observation. Questions focus on the literature, particularly topics presented in the preceding classes, data from preceding sessions or the expertise of the instructor, or anticipation of how the child or their parent might react to the planned session. Through these discussions the instructor focuses the student observations on the relevant learning outcomes. Immediately following the demonstration clinic students are asked to summarize their observations, reflect on the issues of EBP that have arisen within the session and suggest planning for the next session. Subsequent teaching hours use the clinical case as a pivot for discussion of academic content. Through the use of a "live" case, students are exposed to day-to-day EBP issues with real emotional, social, and theoretical considerations needing to be balanced with the research evidence and resource and skill exigencies.

Case-based assessment.   Assessment drives learning (Biggs, 2003), and therefore our assessment tasks are also case based. Across the curriculum this include use of detailed cases for assignments, use of viva voce exams where students are provided with case materials prior to the exam so that they can prepare for the specific case, and modification of exam questions from straight knowledge-based to case-based short-answer questions.

In the example of using a detailed case around which an assignment is based, students in one subject work over many weeks with the progressively revealed material from a complex case. Students submit assessable work on a regular schedule, which is then marked and returned. The next piece of work is not due until the previous has been returned, allowing students to correct misunderstandings before new work is submitted. This cumulative, formative approach to assessment allows both learner and instructor to gauge progress and to rapidly remedy mislearning.

CBL commences in the first year of the undergraduate program where students face case-based exam questions and assignments. For example, in a first-year subject about human communication development a non-case-based exam question might be:

> During the 6 stages of Piaget's sensorimotor period of cognitive development

children learn cognitive antecedents of language development (such as symbolic play). Name two more cognitive antecedents of language development; *briefly* describe what they are and when they begin to emerge.

Such questions have been replaced by case-based questions such as:

Your neighbor's toddler is "furniture creeping," can lift himself to stand, sit unaided, gesture hello and goodbye, understands about 30 words, and uses vocalizations such as "bamigatoo" which sounds like a sentence. He wants to feed himself but often misses his mouth with the food. How old do you think this child is and why?

These CBL assessment tasks encourage students to think about and apply their theoretical knowledge in a clinical context, thus facilitating the transfer of knowledge (Segers, Martens, & Van den Bossche, 2008). This constructive alignment of learning and assessment is EBP in higher education practice (Boud & Falchikov, 2006).

Evaluation

Student evaluation of CBL. CBL is a relatively new way of teaching EBP at the University of Sydney, and therefore we do not yet have end-of-course evaluations to report. These data are being collected and will be presented in the future. However, in subject-specific survey responses since the introduction of CBL, student feedback has been predominantly positive. To use the Voice Sciences and Disorders subject as an example, student comments generally reflect one of four perspectives: (a) no response, (b) positive comment, (c) positive comment about case-based teaching but negative about structure, teaching, or resources, and (d) negative comments. The spread of these

Table 1. Changes in student comments about CBL over two years

Comments	Year	
	2007	2008
Positive comments only	31	49
Positive comments with suggestions for improvements in teaching	38	0
Negative comments	5	4
No comments on CBL	25	46

comments changed over the first two years of using a CBL approach. Data on student comments are shown in Table 1.

Examples of positive student comments about CBL included:

"Teaching incorporated lots of case-based and interactive learning which helped me learn effectively which was complemented by lecture based materials. Very hands on learning."

"Not only did we learn the material but were also given the opportunity to 'be the clinician' and apply what we learned."

"The case-based approach really helped me remember the content."

"I really liked the case based format of the course and I learned a lot more than if it was didactic."

Generally students who made this type of comment rated the course as being an effective way of learning. However, in the first year of implementation, when the instructor was still finding her feet with CBL, students also provided advice on how to improve their learning opportunities.

"Good case-based structure. Perhaps a bit more structured i.e. refer to lecture notes at the same time."

"Case-based study helped learning but maybe more balance with theory; often felt that we lacked direction."

In the second year, after the instructor had engaged in clearer development of learning objectives and scaffolding activities

(Choi & Lee, 2008), student comments were more positive with no suggestions for improvement. This suggests that the CBL is enhanced by reference to theoretical models that provide structure and guidance. The conscious guided use of cases to achieve specific learning outcomes, using appropriate resources and detailed planning and curriculum development, is important in the application of the CBL approach.

Some students have found adapting to a new model of learning and teaching difficult, especially where discovery learning within the context of a case clearly left them feeling uncertain. These students commented negatively about CBL.

"I found it hard to study."

"I did not enjoy the case based learning & group work in voice. It did not seem to be teaching me a lot."

"It has been hard to adapt to case based lectures as it feels like structure sometimes disappears however the instructor taught logically & realistically to prepare us for clinic."

Over time it will be interesting to examine the preferred learning styles and approaches of students in relation to their attitudes to and success with CBL. Additionally students have not directly commented on EBP in relation to CBL, and therefore this will be a focus of future reflection and evaluation.

Instructor evaluation of CBL. Although CBL has obvious benefits in providing students with a framework from which to implement EBP, there are also benefits for academic staff. Arguably the most salient has been the opportunity for instructors to demonstrate their own clinical reasoning in working through the cases with students. As one instructor stated, *"I feel like a clinician again."* Additionally, instructors report that CBL is a much more interesting approach to teaching. *"The richness of the cases and the interaction with the students means that every time it is taught different discussions and decisions occur keeping the material fresh. The student's involvement in the cases is stimulating to me as I teach it."*

"It is very different in terms of teaching. The students are involved in decision making from the first five minutes of the lectures. Theory is taught based on student needs for the case not what I think the students should learn."

Class discussions provide instructors with a clear picture of the students' comprehension in real time. Consequently, instructors can modify their presentation of material, reiterate key points, or provide further explanation, without laboring on less complex issues unnecessarily. The outcome for staff and students has been the creation of a more dynamic and efficient learning environment than had been achieved previously.

CBL appears to foster deep learning (Prosser & Trigwell, 1999). Students engage with materials using their emerging base of knowledge, skills, and clinical experience. The first time undergraduate students encounter a case they approach it with little more than their life experience and their secondary education. At this point, instructors can withhold complex content until students develop foundation knowledge and skills in the topic area. By graduation, students approach cases from a highly analytical perspective, applying all of their previous learning in addressing multiple and confounding issues. The use of CBL, therefore, means that instructors can engage students at any stage of their degree in meaningful real-life clinical scenarios, which provide an ideal platform from which to explore and apply principles of EBP.

"I wanted to know what happened to the case in the long term, did they live happily ever after?"

Additionally CBL activities appear to be highly engaging and motivating to students and instructors. The enthusiasm generated through the use of relevant and meaningful materials, which enables students to project their thinking from the classroom to clinical contexts, generates momentum in the classroom. By encouraging transfer to clinical settings CBL facilitates deep learning, which is supported by student comments and clinically observed behaviors:

"I saw a case similar to the one we did in class so I knew where to start."

One clinical educator reported students saying: *"Oh, that's just like George"* (name of a case) when making a clinical observation of a patient.

Nevertheless, the transition from didactic teaching to CBL has not always been an easy process. Most instructors grappled with the perceived challenge of how to fit all of their old content into a small number of new cases.

"The hardest transition to make was accepting that I didn't have to present ALL of the content. Rather, I needed to present a clear clinical process that was applied to each of the cases, and then encourage the students to use available resources to acquire and consolidate their knowledge."

However, as both instructors and students grew in confidence with the new approach to learning, concerns about not covering all the necessarily content abated.

"I initially fell into the trap of using too many cases but soon realized that as the students became more confident they were more prepared to use the resources and information available and could more easily apply newly acquired knowledge to each of the cases."

The use of CBL can create anxiety for some students, particularly those who prefer didactic teaching. This can, in turn, create difficulties for instructors when students feel challenged by the model of emergent learning employed rather than the traditional explicit presentation of content. Students who feel uncomfortable with CBL may find it difficult to engage productively with peers and instructors in class, and those who self-describe as "perfectionists" may experience anxiety when dealing with case scenarios where there is rarely only one right answer. Therefore, instructors need to be skilled in identifying and supporting students who are struggling with the CBL approach.

The development of a well-constructed and critically aligned curriculum has placed substantial demands on staff. As instructors we have encountered a number of specific challenges in their development of the CBL curriculum including (a) difficulties finding appropriate cases, (b) delays due to the lengthy process of obtaining informed consent from clients, (c) the time it takes to collect, copy, de-identify, and scan case materials, and (d) delays due to technical support issues around uploading audio and video recordings and establishing student access. The use of CBL requires very clear and focused planning and resource development if the desired learning outcomes are to be achieved by students. This process cannot be rushed and would be difficult to achieve without strong support from senior staff and peers.

From student end-of-course surveys in the pre-CBL curriculum we know our graduates feel confident with EBP but have a confused understanding of what it actually involves. We hope that the adoption of CBL will reduce this confusion and promote an increasing ease with EBP in the workplace, leading to a cycle of continuous improvement and lifelong learning. Additionally we anticipate increased speed in moving from novice to entry level as clinicians with consequent flow on in terms of clinical placements and employment prospects.

SUMMARY

Case-based learning appears to have real benefits to students and teachers alike. These appear to include deep learning with EBP being embedded within all aspects of the curriculum, easier transfer of learning from classroom to clinic, renewed interest in learning and teaching for instructors, and the clear enunciation of relevance of research literature to clinical practice for student speech pathologists.

Over time we intend to examine whether our graduating speech pathologists are more comfortable with EBP and are using EBP more effectively than graduates of non-CBL programs. If this occurs then these clinicians will be able to provide best practice throughout their careers leading to better client outcomes.

ACKNOWLEDGMENTS

The authors would like to thank their past and present colleagues in the Discipline of Speech Pathology and the Faculty of Veterinary Science at The University of Sydney for their commitment to the development of case-based learning in the Speech Pathology programs.

Declaration of interest: The authors report no conflicts of interest. The authors alone are responsible for the content and writing of the paper.

REFERENCES

Biggs, J. (2003). *Teaching for quality learning at university. What the student does* (2nd ed.). Philadelphia: SHRE and Open University Press.

Boud, D., & Falchikov, N. (2006). Aligning assessment with long-term learning. *Assessment and Evaluation in Higher Education, 31,* 399–413.

Brackenbury, T., Burroughs, E., & Hewitt, L. E. (2008). A qualitative examination of current guidelines for evidence-based practice in child language intervention. *Language, Speech, and Hearing Services in Schools, 39,* 78–88.

Choi, I., & Lee, K. (2008). A case-based learning environment design for real-world classroom management problem solving. *Technology Trends, 52,* 26–31.

Eliot, T. S. (1950). *The Cocktail Party.* London: Faber & Faber.

Ericksen, S. C. (1984). *The essence of good teaching.* San Francisco: Jossey-Bass.

Fineout-Overholt, E., Stilwell, S. B., & Kent, B. (2008). Teaching EBP through problem-based learning. *Worldviews on Evidence Based Nursing, 5,* 205–207.

Finucane, P., Shannon, W., & McGrath, D. (2009). The financial costs of delivering problem-based learning in a new, graduate-entry medical programme. *Medical Education, 43,* 594–598.

Gillam, S. L., & Gillam, R. B. (2006). Making evidence-based decisions about child language intervention in schools. *Language, Speech, and Hearing Services in Schools, 37,* 304–315.

Gillam, S. L., & Gillam, R. B. (2008). Teaching graduate students to make evidence based intervention decisions. *Application of a seven step process within an authentic learning context. Topics in Language Disorders, 28,* 212–238.

Goldstein, B. A. (2008). Integration of evidence-based practice into the University Clinic. *Topics in Language Disorders, 28,* 200–211.

Kim, S., Phillips, W. R., Pinsky, L., Brock, D., Phillips, K., & Keary, J. (2006). A conceptual framework for developing teaching cases: A review and synthesis of the literature across disciplines. *Medical Education, 40,* 867–876.

Knowles, M., Holton III, E. F., & Swanson, R. A. (2005). *The adult learner: The definitive classic in adult education and human resource development* (6th ed.). Houston, TX: Gulf Publishing Company.

Lincoln, M., & McCabe, P. (2005). Values, necessity and the mother of invention in clinical education. *Advances in Speech Language Pathology, 7,* 153–157.

Metcalfe, C., Lewin, R., Wisher, S., Perry, S., Bannigan, K., & Klaber Moffett, J. (2001). Barriers to implementing the evidence base in four NHS therapies. *Physiotherapy, 87,* 433–440.

O'Connor, S., & Pettigrew, C. M. (2009). The barriers perceived to prevent the successful implementation of evidence-based practice by speech and language therapists. *International Journal of Language & Communication Disorders, 44,* 1018–1035.

Pain, K., Magill-Evans, J., Darrah, J., Hagler, P., & Warren, S. (2004). Effects of profession and facility type on research utilization by rehabilitation professionals. *Journal of Allied Health, 33,* 3–9.

Pennington, L., Roddam, H., Burton, C., Russell, I., Godfrey, C., & Russell, D. (2005). Promoting research use in speech and language therapy: A cluster randomized controlled trial to compare the clinical effectiveness and costs of two training strategies. *Clinical Rehabilitation, 19,* 387–397.

Prosser, M., & Trigwell, K. (1999). *Understanding learning and teaching: The experience in higher education.* Buckingham, UK: Society for Research into Higher Education & Open University Press.

Rybarczyk, B. J., Baines, A. T., McVey, M., Thompson, J. T., & Wilkins, H. (2007). A case-based approach increases student learning outcomes. *Biochemistry and Molecular Biology Education, 35,* 181–186.

Sackett, D. L., Rosenberg, W. M., Gray, J. A., Haynes, R. B., & Richardson, W. S. (1996). Evidence based medicine: What it is and what it isn't. *British Medical Journal, 312*, 71–72.

Segers, M., Martens, R., & Van den Bossche, P. (2008). Understanding how a case-based assessment instrument influences student teachers' learning approaches. *Teaching and Teacher Education: An International Journal of Research and Studies, 24*, 1751–1764.

Speech Pathology Australia. (2001). *Competency-based occupational standards for Speech Pathology (Entry-Level).*

Melbourne, Australia: Speech Pathology Association of Australia.

Togher, L., Lincoln, M., McCabe, P., Munro, N., Power, E., Yiannoukas, C., et al. (2009). *Facilitating the integration of evidence based practice into speech pathology curricula: A scoping study to examine the congruence between academic curricula and work based needs* [Report to the Australian Learning and Teaching Council]. Retrieved July 22, 2009, from http://www.altc.edu.au/resource-facilitating-integration-sydney-2009.

Evidence-based Communication Assessment and Intervention
2009, 3(4), 220–231

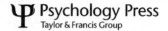

Ψ Psychology Press
Taylor & Francis Group

Building speech-language pathologist capacity for evidence-based practice: A unique graduate course approach

Janet L. Proly & Kimberly A. Murza
University of Central Florida, Department of Communication Sciences and Disorders, Orlando, FL, USA

Abstract

A speech-language pathology graduate-level course using the systematic review and meta-analytic process as a learning tool is described. The course design, content, activities, and pedagogical methods are discussed in depth. Three groups of students worked collaboratively to produce three systematic reviews in the area of language and literacy. This course provided a framework for the completion of the reviews and the development of the students as expert consumers of research. It is suggested that this course framework be used as a tool for building speech-language pathologist capacity in the use of evidence-based decision making.

Keywords: *Evidence-based practice; Speech-language pathology; Graduate; Systematic review; Instruction.*

The ability to critically evaluate the quality of evidence supporting practice is vital to the 21st-century speech-language pathologist (SLP). The American Speech-Language-Hearing Association (ASHA) advocates the clinician's use of the best scientific evidence available, integrated with both the SLP's clinical expertise and the values and needs of the client (American Speech-Language-Hearing Association, 2005). ASHA currently supports this position by conducting systematic reviews and by creating clinical practice guidelines for SLPs and audiologists. Another necessary skill for SLPs working with a diverse clientele is authentic experiences in collaborating with colleagues of varied professional backgrounds and expertise (American Speech-Language-Hearing

Association, 1991). The education of clinicians at both master's and doctoral levels should incorporate these skills to encourage SLPs in providing high-quality and scientifically based practice.

This article's aim is to discuss the systematic review and meta-analytic process as a learning tool for building SLP capacity to implement evidence-based practice (EBP) in their professional caseload. A description of a graduate-level course in EBP in which master and doctoral level students worked collaboratively to produce three systematic reviews that focused on language and literacy serves as a framework.

Why use EBP?

Though EBP is advocated by ASHA, clinicians may question its relevance to their daily practices. However, most SLPs want the best for their clients and strive to ensure that the practices they are using not only work

For correspondence: Janet L. Proly or Kimberly A. Murza, University of Central Florida, Department of Communication Sciences and Disorders, HPA2-Ste 101, 4000 Central Florida Blvd., Orlando, FL 32826, USA. E-mail: jproly@mail.ucf.edu or kimberly.murza@gmail.com

Source of funding: No source of funding reported.

DOI: 10.1080/17489530903432383

but also do no harm. Expert opinion and clinical experience are useful when understood in a scientifically supported context. However, opinion and experience can also result in a clinical bias that may make sense theoretically and logically but not translate into effective practice. To inform practice, SLPs must not only use available evidence, but be well equipped to evaluate the quality and relevance of that evidence. Graduate programs preparing 21st-century SLPs are charged with providing students experiences in critically evaluating treatment research. The systematic review process lends itself to a unique learning opportunity in gathering, evaluating, and synthesizing evidence.

Systematic reviews versus literature reviews

Often, systematic reviews are mistaken for the commonly used narrative literature reviews. However, there are a number of critical distinctions that should be made (e.g., Schlosser & Goetze, 1992). First, literature reviews often neglect to report the manner in which studies were gathered. This is problematic in a number of ways. For example, the reader does not know whether the included studies represent all of the research available on the given topic, only the most convenient evidence available, or those studies that support a particular point of view. Commonly, narrative literature reviewers will search easily accessible databases such as ERIC or PsycINFO, often ignoring the unpublished or grey literature. Additionally, it is generally accepted that studies with positive results are published more often than those with neutral or negative results (Song, Eastwood, Gilbody, Duley, & Sutton, 2000). Without attention to all available evidence both published and unpublished, the narrative review poses the possibility of drawing biased and unfounded conclusions of treatment effectiveness. The application of any conclusions drawn from the narrative review under these conditions

is that the clinician may not be able to determine whether the practice being investigated is relevant to the client or caseload.

At a more advanced level of narrative review, the author may use a method of assessing the viability of the study for conducting a quantitative summary of the results of the included studies. For example, if the reviewer reports the statistical impact of the intervention using the p-value results, the summary is often referred to as a vote-counting approach. In this approach the studies' outcomes are compiled based only on reported levels of significance (i.e., $p < .05$). To illustrate, if a reviewer found five studies on a given topic, she may find that three of the studies revealed positive and significant outcomes (e.g., $p < .05$), and two studies revealed statistically nonsignificant outcomes ($p > .05$). Using the vote-counting approach, the reviewer might conclude that the data support the treatment under study as an effective procedure. The weakness of this approach is that the method ignores critical elements in interpreting the magnitude of effect. Specifically, the vote-counting approach does not account for factors such as sample size, sample heterogeneity, pretreatment effects, and so on, and in fact assumes that significance translates directly to a measure of effectiveness.

The goal of a systematic review is to be transparent, replicable, and documentable in the process of collection, summary, analysis, and interpretation of the available evidence (Chalmers, 2003; Nye, Schwartz, & Schlosser, 2008), resulting in the reduction of reviewer bias. The systematic review objectively considers evidence based on its quality and relevance to the topic area as judged by predetermined information retrieval, data extraction, data analysis/synthesis, and interpretation. From a pedagogical point of view, the process of conducting a systematic review provides an authentic experience to students in searching, evaluating, and interpreting evidence, a skill we believe is increasingly critical for an effective 21st-century SLP.

THE SYSTEMATIC REVIEW PROCESS AS AN EBP GRADUATE COURSE

In an effort to build SLP capacity in EBP techniques, a unique concept was framed in an EBP graduate class at the University of Central Florida (UCF). This unique concept, incorporating lecture as well as cooperative learning and peer-facilitated approaches to learning, sought to teach both master's and doctoral-level students about EBP as they learned how to conduct a systematic review. Although the course had been offered twice before, this offering was the first to include doctoral students in communication sciences and disorders. Building upon previous course offerings, this third offering included several modifications to enhance instruction, content, and student involvement. First, professors assessed the strengths and weaknesses of the past course offerings in terms of student motivation, topic relevance, and time demands for completion. From this analysis, the professors ascertained that student motivation toward the review topic had a substantial influence on the project outcome. That is, success in the course was believed to be related to the students' interest in the review topic independent of the review process.

Secondly, rather than allowing students to select topics ad infinitum, a set of potential topics were presented from which students could choose. The advance determination of potential topics resulted in a more rapid immersion of the students in the individual systematic review than in previous course offerings. Since the doctoral program at UCF has a strong focus on language and literacy, review topics that centered on language and literacy constituted most of the topic choices. The topics chosen were: (a) story grammar instruction to improve narrative comprehension and production in children; (b) does storybook reading increase vocabulary skills in at-risk preschoolers?; and (c) graphic organizer use with elementary through postsecondary students for reading comprehension of expository text.

Third, prior to the beginning of the course, each doctoral student participated in the selection of their topics, while the participating master's-level students were assigned to topics and given the role of review team members. The doctoral students were assigned the role of team leader for their group and were responsible for engaging all members of the group in the review process.

Finally, the potential for presentations of a finished product at international, national, state, and local professional meetings was discussed. Professors encouraged all students, especially the doctoral students, to pursue this professional development opportunity as a means to become engaged in scholarly work, participate in the peer-reviewed presentation submission process, and develop their curriculum vitae. Additionally, students were required to engage in the publication process by registering their topic title with the Education Coordinating Group of the Campbell Collaboration: (http://www.campbellcollaboration.org).

INSTRUCTIONAL FRAMEWORK

The instructional framework for the course included an implicit pedagogical focus, an explicit instructional purpose, and a focus on developing skills to become critical consumers of research. From a pedagogical perspective, the instructional design of the course resembled constructivism, although not explicitly stated by professors, and was exemplified by scaffolded knowledge building, active and authentic learning, and

Table 1. Similarities of steps in original research and systematic review

Steps	Original research	Systematic review
Formulate	Research question	Review objective
Inclusion	Participant characteristics	Study characteristics
Locate	Participants for study	Potential studies meeting inclusion criteria
Select	Participants for study	Studies meeting predefined inclusion criteria
Assess quality	Pretest performance level	Assess the scientific merits of the included studies
Extract data	Implement the experimental condition	Implement a coding process to quantify the important characteristics of the study
Data analysis	Assess the performance based on dependent measures	Assess the impact of treatment based on dependent variable measures
Interpret	Provide analysis of data analysis	Provide analysis of data analysis

learning from one another (Good & Brophy, 2008). The instructional purpose of the course was to conduct a systematic review in order to:

(a) develop an in-depth understanding of intervention research design;
(b) begin to understand the clinical implications of EBP;
(c) develop analytical skills to assess the quality of research evidence;
(d) foster project management skills needed to manage the systematic review process;
(e) provide experience in leadership for the SLP doctoral students.

The skills needed to become critical consumers of research parallel those skills necessary to conduct a systematic review in many ways. Table 1 presents a descriptive summary of the similarities of the scientific methodology associated with original and systematic review research.

These steps were taught throughout the semester and were designed to benefit students conducting a review as well as to assist them in applying their research consumer skills to their coursework, clinical training, and practice. Students who wished

to continue with the systematic review following the completion of the semester were encouraged to do so, but those who did not continue were not penalized. Ultimately, these activities increased student knowledge and led to student publication and presentation opportunities.

Initial conversations among students and professors established the understanding that the systematic review process is lengthy and would likely extend beyond the 15-week semester. As such, the course goal of generating and submitting a Campbell Collaboration title registration and protocol within the 15-week semester time-frame was established. Each group successfully developed and submitted their title registration and protocols within the semester framework. Of the original nine enrolled students, six continued on to complete a systematic review after the course semester ended.

A number of presentations and publications resulted from this and previous EBP course offerings. Between 2005 and 2009 over 15 presentations were made at international, national, and state professional association meetings. In addition, three manuscripts were published in peer-reviewed journals with students serving as either senior or coauthors. This level of student scholarship is certainly recognized as above average for graduate-level students.

AN EIGHT-STEP SYSTEMATIC REVIEW PROCESS

The systematic review process used in the course consisted of the following eight steps:

(1) Formulate a review question.
(2) Define exclusion and inclusion criteria.
(3) Locate studies.
(4) Select studies.
(5) Assess study quality.
(6) Extract data.
(7) Analyze and present results.
(8) Interpret results.

These concepts were covered in depth during weekly three-hour class periods and provided a foundational basis for conducting the systematic review. These eight steps are discussed below in the context of the course's instructional framework, which included (a) systematic information retrieval, (b) quality assessment, (c) data analysis and synthesis, (d) data interpretation, and (e) framing evidence-based clinical decision making.

Systematic information retrieval

Step 1: Formulate a review question. Once students had identified interest areas in the area of language and literacy, the interest areas were explored in terms of relevance to SLP clinical practice contribution as well as for existing research. This exploration included class discussion regarding the abundance or dearth of research support for SLP instructional techniques and practices currently employed in the field. Furthermore, published meta-analyses from various individuals, institutions, organizations, and funding sources were located through electronic database searches and

were discussed in terms of (a) their contribution to SLP language and literacy practices, (b) potential bias generated by the funding source, and (c) needs areas yet to be addressed. From this exploration, three search domain components were devised for investigation: (a) type of intervention, (b) population of interest, and (c) desired outcomes. These three components were framed into a research question that formed the basis for the process of systematic information retrieval. Each group worked together to develop an initial research question and presented it in class for peer editorial comment. Through discussion, revisions were made to each of the groups' questions so that they clearly and succinctly addressed the objective of their reviews.

Step 2: Define exclusion and inclusion criteria. Once a clear review objective was defined, the next step was to establish a priori the criteria that would be used to include or exclude potential studies for the review. The criteria were typically related to the research design (e.g., experimental and quasi-experimental designs), population characteristics (e.g., age, socioeconomic status, race/ethnicity, etc.), intervention characteristics (e.g., minimum length of intervention program, type of intervention, etc.), and outcome characteristics (e.g., achievement, vocabulary, etc.).

The components identified for investigation became part of the eligibility criteria for the systematic review process. One of the tasks for each review team was to develop a coding form that would be used to identify all of the design, participant, intervention, and outcome characteristics reported in each study. In addition, a companion codebook was developed to define key terms and definitions for each component of the coding form used in the data extraction step. An extended description or the coding form and codebook use in this process is provided in the discussion of Step 5 below.

Step 3: Locate studies. The information retrieval process is the strategy used to obtain both the published and unpublished research eligible for inclusion in the review. Several authors (Cooper, 1998; Hunt, 1997; Meline, 2006; Mohr et al., 2000) point out that one of the marks of a high-quality systematic review is the clear presentation of the procedures used by the reviewers to identify and retrieve potential studies for inclusion.

As mentioned above, the search strategy should be transparent and easily reproducible. Having a clear understanding of the components one is examining prior to beginning the search process is essential for documenting the process. Dennis and Abbott (2006) suggested documenting the information retrieval at all stages and including: (a) search terms used, (b) sources used, (c) dates searches run, (d) citations identified from each source, and (e) careful documentation of truncation symbols used and combinations of words used within the various databases. The documentation of this information helps lend credibility to one's approach and helps others appraise the study's value to the question posed.

Once the transparency of the eligibility criteria for the groups' search process was complete and they had devised a plan for documenting their work, the focus shifted to implementing the search strategy. The groups determined the electronic databases and hand searches to be conducted by: (a) investigating past literature on the respective topics, professor recommendations, databases recommended by the Campbell Collaboration, and consultation with an information retrieval expert either at the university or from the Campbell Collaboration. Grey literature, including dissertations and conference presentations, was deemed important by all groups and was included when devising each of the search strategies. A library information specialist, who was an invited class speaker, provided information for conducting the electronic searches including: (a) key databases to consider based on subject area, (b) years indexed by database, (c) thesaurus terms for locating search term synonyms by database, (d) truncation symbols and special characters used to refine searches within each database, (e) availability of specific electronic data bases within the state, (f) electronic citation management software for organizing search results, (g) the possibility of duplication of results from database sources, and (h) how to manage this through citation software.

Professors provided literature support for the methods discussed by the library information specialist as well as other important considerations in the search process. Specifically, reading assignments, in-class exercises, and homework were assigned using the works of Cooper (1998), Dennis and Abbott (2006), Meline (2006), and Torgerson (2003). Students used citation management software including Refworks and Endnote to store their electronic searches. Additionally, each group used a series of GoogleDocs spreadsheets as a central space to track the search and coding process.

Step 4: Select studies. Once the search strategy was developed, each group began the process of conducting the database searches. Each retrieved title was screened for relevance to the review questions. Those titles that were clearly irrelevant were excluded at this level. Any titles that were determined to be potentially relevant to the review were then screened at the abstract level. Full texts of studies were obtained if the study could not be excluded at the abstract level. All screening decisions were based on the inclusion/exclusion criteria described above in Step 2.

Quality assessment of study characteristics

Step 5: Assess study quality. Once the determination was made as to which studies met all the criteria for inclusion in the review, attention turned to the assessment of methodological quality that included components of internal and external validity. Significant class time was spent in presenting the varying dimensions of quality because these are key distinctions to make in the systematic review process and later data analysis (Moberg-Mogren & Nelson, 2006). Class assignments included trial coding of studies that possessed significant positive or negative quality attributes such as type of design (randomized controlled trial, RCT; quasi-experimental; etc.) blinding (single, double, etc), randomization procedure (computer generated, coin flip, etc.), attrition (differential, nondifferential, etc.), or type of analysis (intention-to-treat, assignment–analysis mismatch, etc.).

These and other components contributing to the quality of the studies, especially internal validity threats, were discussed at length. As Torgerson (2003) states, "Although RCTs are widely regarded as the 'gold standard' of effectiveness research, clearly their results are more reliable when the trials are of high quality" (p. 52). Randomized control trials are highly regarded due to their strong internal validity. Torgerson recommends evaluating the internal validity of RCTs based on the following modified characteristics from the Consolidated Standards for Reporting Trials (CONSORT statement; Altman, 1996): (a) concealed randomization, (b) similar attrition rates, (c) no baseline imbalance, (d) blinded or masked follow-up, and (e) sample size.

Additionally, Law and Plunkett (2006) stressed the importance of critically appraising (a) the research question in terms of clarity, appropriate design, and contribution to literature as well as (b) statistical and clinical relevance of outcomes. External validity, or the generalizability of the results, was also a consideration in assessing study quality. Important external validity considerations were discussed in terms of: (a) intervention characteristics (length of the program, number of sessions, and length of sessions, etc.); (b) participant characteristics (age, race/ethnicity, socioeconomic status, setting, grade, etc.); and (c) outcome characteristics: nature of measurement (standardized, criterion referenced, time of postintervention measurement, etc.).

The students in the class synthesized the information regarding methodological quality issues and developed a plan of action toward their respective topics. Two of the three reviews conducted by the students included only RCT studies, the highest quality design. The third review also included quasi-experimental designs but differentiated between the two in the coding process and in the meta-analysis. This third review allowed the designation of study design to be used for comparing RCTs with quasi-experimental designs in determining whether the rigor of the study affected the outcomes. In addition, the instructors discussed the various randomization procedures and how to determine whether a study in fact used a random assignment procedure. This lesson was an important one as the students encountered quite a few studies that labeled themselves as RCTs but after a thorough review the students discovered that some aspect of the random assignment procedure was compromised and therefore categorized the study as a quasi-experimental design. Perhaps the most common example of this was the situation in which a study randomly assigned intact groups, such as classrooms, but analyzed the data at the individual student level. These variations in methodology were recorded on the coding form and accounted for in the meta-analysis.

Data analysis and synthesis

Step 6: Extract data. A major course assignment was the development of a coding form and code-book specific to each group's topic, research question, and inclusion/exclusion criteria. The instructors provided both electronic and hard copy versions of coding forms used in previous reviews that served as guides for the current reviews. Once the coding form was developed, a trial run was conducted using a seminal work in each group's area. The professors and students in each group coded the study independently and then reconciled coding differences through a summary discussion. Ultimately, each coding form was revised to ensure that all vital study characteristics were captured within the form.

The development of the codebook followed a similar process as the coding form and proved to be essential in the coding process as it defined each of the components of the coding form with definitions of key concepts. For instance, a group's definition of a graphic organizer became very important when sifting through the research. Their codebook definition of a graphic organizer required that the graphic organizer contain text. This precise definition excluded some studies that used graphic representations without text, but allowed each coder to accurately exclude those studies based on the definition in the codebook.

Finally, each included full-text study was independently coded by two of the students using a coding form created in the course. An independent third party resolved discrepancies in coding-form responses of the two student coders. A number of studies were excluded during the coding process at both the reconciliation and third-party stages.

Step 7: Analyze and present results. As a complement to the systematic review strategy and quality assessment of study characteristic instruction, the professors provided a foundation in the computation and interpretation of effect sizes. "'Effect size' is simply a way of quantifying the size of the difference between two groups" (Coe, 2002, p. 1). Turner and Bernard (2006) further describe the effect size as "an *estimate* of an intervention's relative effect in the population from which the sample was drawn" (p. 46).

The instruction focusing on data analysis and presentation was composed of the necessary background in calculating effect sizes as well as practical application of effect size calculation. Published study examples were used to discuss, illustrate, and practice effect size calculations. Sample spreadsheets of completed meta-analyses were shown to provide the overall framework as to how the effect size calculation would be used to generate results. An assignment requiring hand calculation of effect sizes from actual studies helped to facilitate student learning. During the following class, effect size calculations were compared, and errors were resolved through modeling of the calculation process.

For the purposes of the class and the nature of the studies examined, the standardized mean difference within the *d* index family was used. The formula for the calculation of the "*d index* is the ratio of the difference between the *sample* mean for the intervention group and the *sample* mean for the control (or comparison) group, divided by the [pooled] sample standard deviation" (Turner & Bernard, 2006, p. 44). The traditional formula for the calculation of the *d* value is as follows:

$$d = \frac{\overline{X}_I - \overline{X}_C}{s_{pooled}}$$

where Xe is the sample mean for the intervention group, Xc is the sample mean for the control (or comparison) group, and SDp is the pooled sample standard deviation.

There are several formulae for computing effect sizes depending on the type of original data presentation (Coe, 2002; Turner & Bernard, 2006). In addition to means and standard deviations, data presented as *t* test, *F* test, and *p*-value are among the over 100 formulae available from the computerized statistical software, Comprehensive Meta-Analysis Version 2 (CMA2; Comprehensive Meta-Analysis Version 2; Borenstein, Hedges, Higgins, & Rothstein, 2005) to calculate the effect size *d* value statistic. All calculations for the reviews conducted for the course used this proprietary software to conduct the analysis required.

Data interpretation

Ultimately, the purpose of a systematic review and meta-analysis is to provide practitioners with information regarding the efficacy of interventions. To do this, as discussed in the previous section, effect sizes are calculated for each outcome in the included studies. However, the researcher must consider the study variables that could potentially impact the magnitude of the intervention effect to provide an interpretation of effect size that is meaningful for the practitioner. To correctly interpret effect sizes there are a number of factors the instructors felt were important to discuss: (a) the magnitude of effect, (b) the direction of effect, (c) the confidence interval, and (d) methodological quality of the study.

Step 8: Interpret results. As discussed previously, the effect size is a continuous measurement that can be both negative and positive. As the effect size increases it can be interpreted as the impact of the intervention on the treated group when compared to the control group (Nye & Harvey, 2006). The most

commonly cited scale for effect sizes interpretation was described by Cohen (1988) and is the one the instructors also adopted. This scale allows effect sizes to be categorized as (a) small = .20, (b) moderate = .50, and (c) large = .80. Although this scale does not provide exact qualitative values of an effect, it does allow researchers to use common language to describe the intervention effect.

Another important consideration is the direction of effect. There are instances in which the intervention outcome for the treatment group could be smaller than the control and still reflect an effective intervention. In treatments that serve to decrease a behavior such as in stuttering treatments or behavioral treatments for self-injurious behaviors, a negative effect size would actually be considered a positive intervention effect favoring the treatment group reflecting a decrease in negative behaviors. This characteristic of intervention direction and outcome measures must be accounted for when coding studies and when conducting the meta-analysis. The instructors explained the importance of including the "direction of effect" on the coding forms for each review and when entering data into a spreadsheet for the meta-analysis. By designating the direction of effect, studies that seek to decrease a behavior may be synthesized with studies seeking to increase behavior, both directions reflecting an improvement due to the intervention.

However, a positive effect alone does not provide enough information. How large of an effect is large enough? The effect size of any study is an estimate of effect, not an exact and certain measure. This is due to the concept of error variance in the measurement of an outcome. In the calculation of the effect size, *d,* the observed value is best interpreted as a potential effect and not an absolute or true effect. When this observed effect is interpreted in terms of the confidence interval, the interpretation allows for the possibility that the true effect could lie anywhere along that interval. As Nye and Harvey (2006) explain, "the 95% confidence interval represents a range of possible scores that we can accept with a fairly high level of confidence as being achievable on replication of the study" (p. 58).

The interpretation of the confidence interval allows the researcher to determine whether an intervention effect is statistically significant. For example, if a study's observed d value is positive, and the lower limit of its confidence interval is negative, we cannot be certain that, if the study was replicated, the treatment group would do better than the control group. Conversely, if a study's lower and upper limit of the confidence interval was positive it would indicate that in at least 95% of replicated studies the treatment group would outperform the control group.

The meta-analysis or synthesis allows the researcher to aggregate the outcomes of multiple studies to provide an overall estimate of effect. This overall estimate of effect also is displayed with a confidence interval to provide an overall measure of statistical significance. Ultimately, the researcher would look to the confidence interval of the cumulative study effects to make a statement about the statistical significance and overall efficacy of the intervention.

Framing evidence-based clinical decisions

Producing a systematic review should not occur in a vacuum but should inform clinical practice as to the efficacy of an investigated intervention and outcome. Although the course focused on the systematic review process, the instructors also brought the discussion back to the "so what" question. The conclusions of any systematic review should address the "so what" question in terms of the practice of professionals in the field of investigation. ASHA defines the goal of EBP as, "the integration of (a) clinical expertise, (b) best current evidence, and (c) client values to provide high-quality services reflecting the interests, values, needs and choices of the individuals we serve" (American Speech-Language-Hearing Association, 2004, p. 1). Using this definition as a guideline, the practicing SLP would use the systematic review and meta-analysis as one piece of the evidence-based decision-making process. Practicing SLPs not only want to know whether an intervention is effective, but want to know under what circumstances the intervention is most effective and with whom. These questions can be addressed through the analysis of study variables. The study coding process allows the researcher to make comparisons among studies that have similar participants, interventions, dosage, or settings. This information is critical for many reasons including the fact that some interventions may work best for certain age groups or for participants diagnosed with a specific disorder.

Treatment intensity is another variable that is relevant to the practicing clinician. SLPs need to know how to deliver the most efficacious intervention. This question is critical especially for SLPs who work with third-party payers and their accompanying service restrictions (time, cost, location, etc.). SLPs need to know which interventions show the "biggest bang for the buck" regardless of payer source (e.g., schools, government, insurance, private, etc.). SLPs have an ethical obligation to use the best available evidence to make clinical decisions. Although clinical expertise is part of the EBP process it should not be considered the end-all in terms of providing the best services for clients. As Konnerup and Schwartz (2006) suggest, "there is an urgent need to systematically include other forms of knowledge like research findings and summaries" (p. 81). The systematic review and meta-analysis process has the potential of significantly influencing the SLP's ability to make better

EBP decisions and ultimately improving the communication needs of his or her clients.

SUMMARY

Course design, content, and activities had a significant impact on both master's and doctoral graduate students. All students acquired the knowledge and skills necessary to locate, analyze, and critically evaluate existing research. This knowledge is essential to the application of scientific-based evidence in clinical practice, as well as crucial for future investigators to contribute to the existing research base (Dollaghan, 2007). In addition, encouraging doctoral students to accept a leadership role (a) enhanced collaboration among students, (b) afforded doctoral students the opportunity to assume a mentoring role and experience the reality of collaboration, (c) enabled participation in a joint intellectual effort, and (d) honed problem-solving skills in interpersonal relationships and academic endeavors. The doctoral students reported that the course provided the impetus to actively engage in professional activities including: (a) international, national, and state presentations, (b) discerning and creating opportunities for publication and professional development, (c) disseminating and translating research to practice, and (d) publishing research.

ACKNOWLEDGEMENTS

Special thanks to Stacey Pavelko and Jamie Schwartz for their contributions to the conference presentation proposal which served as inspiration for this manuscript. Special thanks to Chad Nye for his helpful comments and time following this manuscript's acceptance.

Declaration of interest: The authors report no conflicts of interest. The authors alone are responsible for the content and writing of this article.

REFERENCES

Altman, D. G. (1996). Better reporting of randomised controlled trials: The CONSORT statement. *British Medical Journal, 313*, 570–571.

American Speech-Language-Hearing Association. (1991). *A model for collaborative service delivery for students with language-learning disorders in the public schools* [Relevant paper]. Available from www.asha.org/policy

American Speech-Language-Hearing Association. (2004). *Evidence-based practice in communication disorders: An introduction* [Technical report]. Available from www.asha.org/policy

American Speech-Language-Hearing Association. (2005). *Evidence-based practice in communication disorders* [Position statement]. Available from www.asha.org/policy

Borenstein, M., Hedges, L., Higgins, J., & Rothstein, H. (2005). *Comprehensive Meta-Analysis Version 2* [Computer software]. Englewood, NJ: Biostat. Retrieved July 01, 2009, from http://www.metaanalysis.com

Chalmers, I. (2003). Trying to do more good than harm in policy and practice: The role of rigorous, transparent, up-to-date evaluations. *The Annals of the American Academy of Political and Social Science, 589*, 22–40.

Coe, R. (September, 2002). *It's the effect size, stupid: What effect size is and why it is important.* Paper presented at the annual conference of the British Educational Research Association, Exeter, UK.

Cohen, J. (1988). *Statistical power analysis for the behavioral sciences* (2nd ed.). Hillsdale, NJ: Lawrence Erlbaum Associates.

Cooper, H. (1998). *Synthesizing research* (3rd ed.). Thousand Oaks, CA: Sage Publications.

Dennis, J., & Abbott, J. (2006). Information retrieval: Where's your evidence? *Contemporary Issues in Communication Science and Disorders, 33*, 11–20.

Dollaghan, C. A. (2007). *The handbook for evidence-based practice in communication disorders.* Baltimore, MD: Paul H. Brookes Publishing Co.

Good, T. L., & Brophy, J. E. (2008). *Looking in classrooms* (10th ed.). Boston, MA: Pearson Education.

Hunt, M. (1997). *How science takes stock: The story of meta-analysis.* New York: Russell Sage Foundation.

Konnerup, M., & Schwartz, J. (2006). Translating systematic reviews into policy and practice: An international perspective. *Contemporary Issues in Communication Science and Disorders, 33*, 79–82.

Law, J., & Plunckett, C. (2006). Grading study quality in systematic reviews. *Contemporary Issues in Communication Science and Disorders, 33*, 28–36.

Meline, T. (2006). Selecting studies for systematic review: Inclusion and exclusion criteria. *Contemporary Issues in Communication Science and Disorders, 33*, 21–27.

Moberg-Mogren, E., & Nelson, D. (2006). Evaluating the quality of reporting occupational therapy randomized controlled trials by expanding the CONSORT criteria. *The American Journal of Occupational Therapy, 60*, 226–235.

Mohr, D., Cook, D. J., Eastwood, S., Olkin, I., Drummond, R., & Stroup, D. F. (2000). *British Journal of Surgery, 354*, 1448–1454.

Nye, C., & Harvey, J. (2006). Interpreting and maintaining the evidence. *Contemporary Issues in Communication Science and Disorders, 33*, 56–60.

Nye, C., Schwartz, J. B., & Schlosser, R. W. (November, 2008). *Systematic reviews & clinical practice: From production to application*. Short course presented at the American Speech-Language-Hearing Association Conference, Chicago, IL.

Schlosser, R. W., & Goetze, H. (1992). Effectiveness and treatment validity of interventions addressing self-injurious behavior: From narrative reviews to meta-analysis. *Advances in Learning and Behavioral Disabilities, 7*, 135–175.

Song, F., Eastwood, A. J., Gilbody, S., Duley, L., & Sutton, A. J. (2000). Publication and related biases. *Health Technology Assessment, 4*, 1–115.

Torgerson, C. J. (2003). *Systematic reviews*. Harrisburg, PA: The Continuum International Publishing Group.

Turner III, H. M., & Bernard, R. M. (2006). Calculating and synthesizing effect sizes. *Contemporary Issues in Communication Science and Disorders, 33*, 42–55.

Evidence-based Communication Assessment and Intervention
2009, 3(4), 232–237

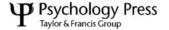

Teaching evidence-based practice in a problem-based learning course in speech-language pathology

Parimala Raghavendra

Division of Research & Innovation, Novita Children's Services, Regency Park, SA, Australia; Department of Speech Pathology & Audiology, Flinders University, Adelaide, SA, Australia; Division of Health Sciences, University of South Australia, Adelaide, SA, Australia

Abstract

This paper presents an innovative approach undertaken to teach evidence-based practice (EBP) in a master's course in speech-language pathology that utilizes problem-based learning (PBL). The workshop content, the assessment task of preparing a critically appraised topic, and students' feedback and reflections demonstrate the strong nexus between the content of EBP, and the teaching approach and PBL format.

Keywords: Teaching evidence-based practice; Problem-based learning; Critically appraised topic.

In Australia, speech-language pathology training programs typically consist of either a four-year undergraduate degree or two-year intensive master's degree. One can enter the profession on graduating from either one of the above programs from an accredited university. Evidence-based practice (EBP) is taught in many university programs that offer undergraduate and master's degrees in speech-language pathology. One such program is the two-year Master of Speech-Language Pathology offered at Flinders University in Adelaide, Australia. This program began in 2006 with an intake of around 18 students. It is unique in Australia in that it does not require specific undergraduate degrees or courses because the intention is to offer an opportunity for career change and contribute to

diversity within the profession. Therefore students have a diverse range of backgrounds including study and often work experience in areas such as teaching, psychology, nursing, finance, or even journalism.

The Flinders University master's course is based on principles designed to encourage lifelong learning, thus incorporating an innovative enquiry-based curriculum utilizing a problem-based learning (PBL) format. Halliwell (2008) summarized key principles of PBL as follows: (a) Students work in small groups exploring practice-based issues usually provided in the form of clinical scenarios; (b) groups set their learning tasks; (c) issues are explored across curricular areas; and (d) practical application drives knowledge acquisition. PBL aims to facilitate knowledge production using information from a range of sources, including various levels of research and clinical evidence.

In the master's program, PBL cases are supported by other teaching and learning

For correspondence: Parimala Raghavendra, Division of Research & Innovation, Novita Children's Services, PO Box 2438, Regency Park, SA 5942, Australia. E-mail: parimala. raghavendra@novita.org.au

Source of funding: No source of funding reported.

http://www.psypress.com/EBCAI   DOI: 10.1080/17489530903399160 strategies, including lectures, practical, and student seminars and presentations. Students experience work-based learning from the beginning, giving them opportunities to integrate knowledge with practice under the supervision of clinical educators. The course also uses a variety of assessment methods including peer and self-assessment and performance within authentic tasks and competency-based assessment of clinical work (COMPASS®, McAllister, Lincoln, Ferguson, & McAllister, 2006).

Within this framework, the author was invited to teach a course on EBP entitled *Research into Practice* at the end of the second year of the master's program. The educational aims of the topic are to: (a) enable students to develop skills in formulating answerable clinical questions and finding and evaluating the research evidence to support and enhance their clinical practice, (b) encourage the development of critical appraisal skills that enable the students to evaluate the quality of their own and other scholars' research, (c) emphasize the importance of integration of client/family values, research evidence with clinical expertise in the diagnosis and treatment of communication and swallowing disorders, (d) apply their knowledge by identifying a clinical question and then evaluating the literature to determine the research evidence to answer the question, and (e) develop skills in oral and written presentation of research findings.

CONTENT

The content for *Research into Practice* was delivered in a workshop format over 3 days with small-group and whole-group sessions addressing issues common to speech-language pathology. The topic assessment involved a written report of and an oral presentation on a critically appraised topic (CAT) or synthesized critically appraised papers (CAPs). McCluskey (2003) describes a CAT as a succinct summary of research evidence on a particular topic usually arising from a clinical issue. The research evidence is from more than one appraised paper, but it is not as rigorous as a systematic review. A CAP, on the other hand, is a critical appraisal and summary of one study or paper (McCluskey, 2003).

PBL is a strategy for facilitating quality learning, which includes devising quality assessment tasks. Boud and Falchikov (2006) argued that in preparing students for lifelong learning, assessment in university education must reflect not only immediate learning requirements but long-term learning as well. They recommend that students need to be able to assess their own learning in a similar way to their approach in highly contextualized environments of work and life. They suggest that assessment should provide opportunities for students to engage with communities of practice rather than just educational staff, foster reflexivity and systematic inquiry, and deal with elements of tasks not fully developed by educational institutions.

The development of a CAT is considered a quality assessment task because it addresses the first three learning objectives of the course. The students are able to participate in determining aspects of the assessment by developing their own clinical question. The task is authentic and relevant to their future practice as they can utilize the knowledge and skills of writing a CAT for any client with communication disorder. The CAT can also be used for a group of clients or in an area of practice. Several students have used their clinical placement and discussions with their supervisors to develop their question, thus involving an extended community beyond their training institution. It is envisaged that the CAT developed by the student could be used in clinical practice after it has been evaluated. Outlined below is a brief overview of the workshop content and guidelines for the development of a CAT.

Day 1 covered the background to EBP including evidence-based medicine and EBP in other fields, myths about EBP, and what EBP means for a client, clinician, service provider, policy maker, researcher, and teacher/lecturer. The next two days were focused on a description and discussion of seven steps to undertake EBP (adapted from Schlosser & Raghavendra, 2003) and practical experience undertaking a few of the steps:

1. *How to ask a clinically relevant and answerable question?* PICO (Patient/population, Intervention, Comparison/control, Outcomes; Richardson, Wilson, Nishikawa, & Hayward, 1995) and PESICO (Person/problem, Environment, Stakeholders, Intervention, Control/comparison, Outcomes; Schlosser, Koul, & Costello, 2007) templates were used, and small group work was utilized in framing clinically relevant answerable questions.

2. *How to search for relevant articles using various databases?* A three-hour hands-on workshop in the university library guided by an experienced librarian was completed. The students had an opportunity to try various databases and learn how to strategically search for research information, which they found to be extremely useful. Since the students had to start thinking about their assignment for the course (developing a CAT) they already had an idea of a clinical question and were able to use the database searches in a meaningful way. The first group of students strongly felt that the knowledge of various databases and skills of searching them efficiently and effectively should be taught at the beginning of their course, as they could use these resources in various PBL and other assignments.

This feedback was adopted for current students who received an orientation to the use of database resources. However, the current students commented that they benefitted from further focused training as it was contextualized. Differences between a systematic review and literature review were also highlighted.

3. *How do you critically appraise research, that is, what do you need to look for in articles?* A significant amount of time was used in exploring this step. Critical appraisal tools (EVIDAAC Systematic Rating Scale, Schlosser et al., 2008; Physiotherapy Evidence Database Scale, PEDro Scale, 1999; McMaster critical appraisal tools, Law et al., 1998; Letts et al., 2007), and hierarchy of evidence in medicine/allied health and a proposed hierarchy for augmentative and alternative communication (Schlosser & Raghavendra, 2004) were introduced and explained. A systematic review was appraised by the group. Articles in various areas of speech-language pathology using different research designs were distributed to the students (e.g., a randomized control trial, systematic review, and cross-sectional, case-control, and single-case experimental designs). The students utilized a weekend to read the articles and appraise the evidence using the appropriate tools. Critical appraisal was undertaken in small groups of three to four students with the whole group coming together after each article. The discussions were predominantly around design issues and clarity of explanations given by authors. Students reflected that even studies using strong designs that control for internal validity by "well-known" researchers had some degree of flaw, and this was a learning experience for them. They kept asking, "Why can't authors use these appraisal tools and design studies around them so that their studies get the higher ratings?" This led to

discussions around the type of question, study design, participant recruitment challenges, resources, participant drop-outs, practical difficulties in designing studies, and journal requirements that restrict the provision of detailed information. Some or all of these factors may contribute to poorer scores on appraisal ratings for articles. A study using qualitative research methodology was also appraised using McMaster critical review form for qualitative studies (Letts et al., 2007).

4. *How do you collate and synthesize evidence?* The definition of a CAT and a CAP and steps taken to complete them were presented as a way to collate and synthesize the research evidence. Differences between a systematic review and a CAT were also examined (Wendt, 2006).

5. *Implementing the evidence in practice.* Developing and using clinical guidelines as one method of implementing EBP were discussed. Examples of guidelines, sources for finding clinical guidelines, and tools to appraise guidelines were presented. Methods to promote the integration of clinical expertise, clients' perspectives, and research evidence were discussed. A practical example of an organizational approach was also shared.

6. *Evaluating the use of the evidence.* The importance of documenting the impact of EBP on practice through systematic data collection from all stakeholders was stressed. Ongoing revisions of a CAT and reviewing clinical guidelines were discussed as ways of evaluating the evidence.

7. *Disseminating the EBP findings.* Since EBP is a relatively new way of providing services, the importance of dissemination of EBP processes and outcomes was

highlighted.

Day 3 covered important issues such as facilitators and barriers to EBP with input from clinical supervisors and other faculty. The journal of *Evidence-based Communication Assessment and Intervention* (EBCAI) was highlighted as a key source of evidence for practitioners and as a facilitator of EBP as "all the hard work has been done" by authors, commentators, and the editors. The workshop concluded with the presentation of different viewpoints on EBP and emphasizing the lifelong learning principles embedded in EBP. All resources are made available to the students on a secure section of the University Web site.

TOPIC REQUIREMENT

As mentioned earlier, each student had to develop a CAT for his or her assessment. Traditionally a CAT is developed by two or more individuals. Due to clinical placement requirements occurring around the time of the EBP course, students could not work in groups to develop a CAT. Thus each student developed a CAT for their clinically relevant question. The following guidelines were given to the students to develop their CAT: First, select an issue/topic area related to a client or clinical setting or an area of their clinical interest. Second, develop a clinically relevant answerable question following the PICO/PESICO template; they were encouraged to use either of the templates depending on the area, as each template had specific advantages. Some students preferred the PICO template as it helped them to be succinct while others commented that the PESICO template helped them to further clarify their question due to incorporating the environment and the various stakeholders' perspectives. Third, use appropriate search terms and search databases for research articles. Fourth, find and obtain at least three articles with the strongest level of evidence, published in journals (a maximum of five articles); students were asked to search for systematic reviews first. Fifth, using Joanna Briggs Institute (2008) Levels of Evidence and Schlosser and Raghavendra's (2004) hierarchy table of evidence, state the level of evidence for each study; students were asked to use both ratings to give them an understanding that the same study design could get slightly varying levels of evidence depending on the hierarchy used. Sixth, use appropriate tools (PEDro, 1999; McMaster critical appraisal tools, Law et al., 1998; Letts et al., 2007) and appraise each article. Seventh, summarize each article and synthesize the findings. Eighth, provide suggestions on how the research evidence can be used in practice. Ninth, give the clinical bottom line.

EVALUATION

The feedback after each day of the workshop was extremely positive. Students commented that the information was presented in an understandable way, and they were learning a new way to analyze and understand the value of research in relation to practice. They wished that they had had the EBP workshop at the start of their master's course so that they could use the skills in all other subjects. It remains a challenge for course planners as to the timing of the course. The students in this course did not have any background knowledge in speech-language pathology, hence may not have been able to understand the relevance or the importance of EBP earlier in the curriculum.

The presence of experienced clinicians and faculty in the workshops made the discussions stimulating as they could provide real-world examples of the importance of EBP and challenges and facilitators for implementing EBP. The students' feedback reflected the need to provide a strong foundation in understanding various research designs and methodology as these were essential in the critical appraisal of research.

The students found developing a CAT to be a complex and challenging task. The critical appraisal aspect and extracting the appropriate information were difficult. Students felt that they really needed more experience in appraising articles. A majority of the students presented the outcomes from their CAT in a succinct manner. Examples of CATs developed included: (a) "Effect of tracheostomy and tracheostomy tubes on aspiration status in adult patients"; (b) "Does dialogic reading promote the development of oral language and emergent literacy skills in preschool children?"; (c) "The effect of oral stimulation/oral support appears effective in improving preterm infants sucking abilities but further research is needed." The future plan is to submit the CATs of students who score above 75% to the EBCAI journal and post CATs of students who score above 65% on to an appropriate Web site.

REFLECTIONS

The teaching of EBP in speech-language pathology is valuable, and the workshop coupled with the CAT assessment tasks effectively supplements the PBL curriculum. EBP education certainly fits within the PBL philosophy of developing critical thinking and the interaction between research evidence, clinical expertise, and practice. The workshop and developing a CAT uses quality teaching and assessment approaches that could be included into any kind of curriculum structure. It is also evident that all subject areas of speech-language pathology need to embrace and include EBP in the course work and topic assessments. However, a stand-alone workshop or tutorial on EBP is imperative. The timing of teaching EBP is a difficult decision. Students need to understand the basic process of communication and communication disorders prior to such a module. They need to be introduced to principles of EBP as early as possible in their course work and then have the concept reiterated in other areas of speech-language pathology such as fluency disorders, aphasia, child language, and augmentative and alternative communication. For this to occur all faculty need to have a thorough knowledge of EBP, be up to date with research evidence in their own fields of expertise, and also understand the clinical issues. The knowledge and skills learned to undertake and implement EBP in speech-language pathology will equip students with tools for lifelong learning. Critical reflection is a key part, and EBP provides a good framework.

ACKNOWLEDGMENTS

I would like to thank Dr. Sue McAllister, Senior Lecturer, and Associate Professors Paul McCormack and Janet Baker, Department of Speech Pathology and Audiology, Flinders University for their input into this paper and support during the teaching of the course.

Declaration of interest: The author reports no conflicts of interest. The author alone is responsible for the content and writing of the paper.

REFERENCES

Boud, D., & Falchikov, N. (2006). Aligning assessment with long-term learning. *Assessment & Evaluation in Higher Education, 31*, 399–413.

Halliwell, V. (2008). Challenging knowledge reproduction: Problem-based learning for evidence-based practice. *British Journal of Occupational Therapy, 71*, 257–259.

Joanna Briggs Institute. (2008). *JBI Levels of Evidence*. Retrieved September 15, 2009, from http://www.joannabriggs.edu.au/pubs/approach.php

Law, M., Stewart, D., Pollock, N., Letts, L., Bosch, J., & Westmorland, M. (1998). *Critical review form—quantitative studies*. Retrieved September 4, 2009, from McMaster University Web site: http://www-fhs.mcmaster.ca/rehab/ebp/pdf/quanreview.pdf

Letts, L., Wilkins, S., Law, M., Stewart, D., Bosch, J., & Westmorland, M. (2007). *Critical review form—qualitative studies (Version 2.0)*. Retrieved September 4, 2009, from McMaster University Web site: http://www.srs-mcmaster.ca/Portals/20/pdf/ebp/qualreview_version2.0.pdf

McAllister, S., Lincoln, M., Ferguson, A., & McAllister, L. (2006). *COMPASS®: Competency assessment in speech-language pathology*. Melbourne, Australia: Speech Pathology Australia.

McCluskey, A. (2003). *Occupational therapy critically appraised topics*. Retrieved September 4, 2009, from http://www.otcats.com/intro.html

PEDro Scale. (1999). *Physiotherapy Evidence Database Scale*. Retrieved November 6, 2009, from http://www.pedro.org.au/english/downloads/pedro-scale/

Richardson, W., Wilson, M., Nishikawa, J., & Hayward, R. (1995). The well-built clinical question: A key to evidence-based decisions. *ACP Journal Club, 123*(3), A12–A13.

Schlosser, R. W., Koul, R., & Costello, J. (2007). Asking well-built questions for evidence-based practice in augmentative and alternative communication. *Journal of Communication Disorders, 40*, 225–238.

Schlosser, R. W., & Raghavendra, P. (2003). Toward evidence-based practice in augmentative and alternative communication. In R. W. Schlosser (Ed.), *The efficacy of augmentative and alternative communication: Toward evidence-based practice* (pp. 259–297). New York: Academic Press.

Schlosser, R. W., & Raghavendra, P. (2004). Evidence based-practice in augmentative and alternative communication. *Augmentative and Alternative Communication, 20*, 1–21.

Schlosser, R. W., Raghavendra, P., Sigafoos, J., Eysenbach, G., Blackstone, S., & Dowden, P. (2008). *EVIDAAC Systematic Review Scale*. Unpublished manuscript, Northeastern University, Boston, MA.

Wendt, O. (2006). *Developing critically appraised topics (CATs)*. Paper presented at the meeting of the American Speech-Language Hearing Association, Division 12: Augmentative and Alternative Communication (DAAC), 7th Annual Conference, San Antonio, TX. Retrieved September 9, 2009, from http://www.edst.purdue.edu/aac/AACpresentations.htm

Evidence-Based Communication Assessment and Intervention
Volume 3, 2009, List of Contents

Issue 2: June

EBP ADVANCEMENT CORNER

Issue 3: September

EDITORIAL

REVIEW-TREATMENT

TREATMENT

Issue 4: December

Special issue: Teaching Evidence-Based Practice, edited by Ralf W. Schlosser and Jeff Sigafoos

INTRODUCTION

SPECIAL ISSUE PAPERS

VOLUME 3 INDEXES

Evidence-Based Communication Assessment and Intervention
Volume 3, 2009, Author Index